T0226957

Concussion in Sports

Editor

SCOTT R. LAKER

PHYSICAL MEDICINE AND REHABILITATION CLINICS OF NORTH AMERICA

www.pmr.theclinics.com

Consulting Editor
SANTOS F. MARTINEZ

May 2016 • Volume 27 • Number 2

ELSEVIER

1600 John F. Kennedy Boulevard ● Suite 1800 ● Philadelphia, Pennsylvania, 19103-2899

http://www.theclinics.com

**PHYSICAL MEDICINE AND REHABILITATION CLINICS OF NORTH AMERICA Volume 27, Number 2
May 2016 ISSN 1047-9651, ISBN 978-0-323-44521-4**

Editor: Jennifer Flynn-Briggs
Developmental Editor: Donald Mumford

Reprints. For copies of 100 or more of articles in this publication, please contact the Commercial Reprints Department, Elsevier Inc., 360 Park Avenue South, New York, NY 10010-1710. Tel.: 212-633-3874; Fax: 212-633-3820; E-mail: reprints@elsevier.com.

Physical Medicine and Rehabilitation Clinics of North America (ISSN 1047-9651) is published quarterly by Elsevier Inc., 360 Park Avenue South, New York, NY 10010-1710. Months of issue are February, May, August, and November. Business and Editorial Offices: 1600 John F. Kennedy Blvd., Suite 1800, Philadelphia, PA 19103-2899. Customer Service Office: 3251 Riverport Lane, Maryland Heights, MO 63043. Periodicals postage paid at New York, NY and additional mailing offices. Subscription price per year is $280.00 (US individuals), $538.00 (US institutions), $100.00 (US students), $335.00 (Canadian individuals), $709.00 (Canadian institutions), $210.00 (Canadian students), $415.00 (foreign individuals), $709.00 (foreign institutions), and $210.00 (foreign students). Foreign air speed delivery is included in all *Clinics* subscription prices. All prices are subject to change without notice. **POSTMASTER:** Send address changes to *Physical Medicine and Rehabilitation Clinics of North America*, Customer Service Office: Elsevier Health Sciences Division, Subscription Customer Service, 3251 Riverport Lane, Maryland Heights, MO 63043. **Customer Service: 1-800-654-2452 (US). From outside of the United States, call 314-447-8871. Fax: 314-447-8029. E-mail: JournalsCustomer Service-usa@elsevier.com (for print support); JournalsOnlineSupport-usa@elsevier.com (for online support).**

Physical Medicine and Rehabilitation Clinics of North America is indexed in *Excerpta Medica, MEDLINE/ PubMed (Index Medicus), Cinahl, and Cumulative Index to Nursing and Allied Health Literature.*

Contributors

CONSULTING EDITOR

SANTOS F. MARTINEZ, MD, MS
Diplomate of the American Academy of Physical Medicine and Rehabilitation, Certificate of Added Qualification Sports Medicine, Campbell Clinic, Assistant Professor, Department of Orthopaedics, University of Tennessee, Memphis, Tennessee

EDITOR

SCOTT R. LAKER, MD
Associate Professor, University of Colorado School of Medicine, Aurora, Colorado

AUTHORS

MICHAEL L. ALOSCO, PhD
Chronic Traumatic Encephalopathy Program, Boston University School of Medicine, Boston, Massachusetts

DAVID A. BAKER, PsyD
Research Associate Professor, UBMD Department of Orthopaedics and Sports Medicine and Nuclear Medicine, Jacobs School of Medicine and Biomedical Sciences; School of Social Work; University at Buffalo, Buffalo, New York

JOHN G. BAKER, PhD
UBMD Department of Orthopaedics and Sports Medicine, SUNY Buffalo Jacobs School of Medicine and Biomedical Sciences, Buffalo, New York

GARNI BARKHOUDARIAN, MD
Pacific Pituitary Disorders Center, John Wayne Cancer Institute, Providence Saint John's Health Center, Santa Monica, California

LEAH G. CONCANNON, MD
Clinical Assistant Professor, Division of Sports and Spine, Department of Rehabilitation Medicine, University of Washington, Seattle, Washington

AMY K. CONNERY, PsyD
Department of Physical Medicine and Rehabilitation, Children's Hospital Colorado, University of Colorado School of Medicine, Aurora, Colorado

GERARD A. GIOIA, PhD
Professor, Department of Pediatrics and Psychiatry and Behavioral Sciences, Division of Pediatric Neuropsychology, Children's National Health System, George Washington University School of Medicine, Rockville, Maryland

CHRISTOPHER C. GIZA, MD
Interdepartmental Programs for Neuroscience and Biomedical Engineering,
Department of Neurosurgery, UCLA Brain Injury Research Center, Semel Institute, David
Geffen School of Medicine at UCLA, Mattel Children's Hospital - UCLA; Interdepartmental
Programs for Neuroscience and Biomedical Engineering, Division of Pediatric Neurology,
Department of Pediatrics, UCLA Brain Injury Research Center, Semel Institute, David
Geffen School of Medicine at UCLA, Mattel Children's Hospital - UCLA, Los Angeles,
California

MICHAEL R. GREHER, PhD, ABPP-CN
Associate Professor, University of Colorado School of Medicine, Department of
Neurosurgery, Academic Office One, Aurora, Colorado

JUSTIN M. HONCE, MD
Assistant Professor, Department of Radiology, University of Colorado School of
Medicine, Aurora, Colorado

DAVID A. HOVDA, PhD
Interdepartmental Program for Neuroscience, Departments of Neurosurgery; Medical
and Molecular Pharmacology, UCLA Brain Injury Research Center, Semel Institute,
David Geffen School of Medicine at UCLA, Los Angeles, California

BERTRAND R. HUBER, MD, PhD
VA Boston HealthCare System; Department of Neurology, Boston University School of
Medicine, Boston, Massachusetts

JOHN HYDEN, MD
Campbell Clinic Orthopaedics, Fellowship Director, Primary Care Sports Medicine
Fellowship, Germantown, Tennessee; University of Tennessee Health Science Center,
Memphis, Tennessee;

GRANT L. IVERSON, PhD
Professor, Department of Physical Medicine and Rehabilitation, Harvard Medical School;
Spaulding Rehabilitation Hospital; MassGeneral Hospital for Children Sport Concussion
Program; Home Base Program, Red Sox Foundation, Massachusetts General Hospital,
Boston, Massachusetts; Department of Physical Medicine and Rehabilitation, Center for
Health and Rehabilitation, Harvard Medical School, Charlestown, Massachusetts

ISAAC JONES, MD
Department of Radiology, University of Colorado School of Medicine, Aurora, Colorado

MICHAEL W. KIRKWOOD, PhD
Department of Physical Medicine and Rehabilitation, Children's Hospital Colorado,
University of Colorado School of Medicine, Aurora, Colorado

SCOTT R. LAKER, MD
Associate Professor, University of Colorado School of Medicine, Aurora, Colorado

JOHN J. LEDDY, MD
Professor, UBMD Department of Orthopaedics and Sports Medicine, SUNY Buffalo
Jacobs School of Medicine and Biomedical Sciences, Buffalo, New York

ANN C. McKEE, MD
VA Boston HealthCare System; Department of Neurology, Boston University School of Medicine; Chronic Traumatic Encephalopathy Program, Boston University School of Medicine; Department of Pathology, Boston University School of Medicine, Boston, Massachusetts

ADELE MERON, MD
Chief Resident, Department of Physical Medicine and Rehabilitation, University of Colorado School of Medicine, Denver, Colorado

MARY MILLER PHILLIPS, MD
Fellow, Brain Injury Medicine, Department of Physical Medicine and Rehabilitation, University of Pittsburgh Medical Center, Pittsburgh, Pennsylvania

LIDIA NAGAE, MD
Assistant Professor, Department of Radiology, University of Colorado School of Medicine, Aurora, Colorado

ERIC NYBERG, MD
Assistant Professor, Department of Radiology, University of Colorado School of Medicine, Aurora, Colorado

ROBIN L. PETERSON, PhD
Department of Physical Medicine and Rehabilitation, Children's Hospital Colorado, University of Colorado School of Medicine, Aurora, Colorado

BENJAMIN PETTY, MD
Campbell Clinic Orthopaedics, Germantown; University of Tennessee Health Science Center, Memphis, Tennessee

CHRISTOPHER RANDOLPH, PhD
Department of Neurology, Loyola University Medical Center, Maywood, Illinois

CARA CAMIOLO REDDY, MD, MMM
Medical Director, Brain Injury Program, Department of Physical Medicine and Rehabilitation, UPMC Rehabilitation Institute, University of Pittsburgh Medical Center, Pittsburgh, Pennsylvania

THOR D. STEIN, MD, PhD
VA Boston HealthCare System; Chronic Traumatic Encephalopathy Program, Boston University School of Medicine; Department of Pathology, Boston University School of Medicine; Bedford Veterans Affairs Medical Center, Bedford, Massachusetts

BARRY WILLER, PhD
Professor, Department of Psychiatry, Jacobs School of Medicine and Biomedical Sciences, University at Buffalo, Buffalo, New York

JULIE WILSON, MD
Assistant Professor, Children's Hospital Colorado, Aurora, Colorado

Contents

> Concussion, or mild traumatic brain injury (TBI), affects millions of patients worldwide. Understanding the pathophysiology of TBI can help manage its repercussions. The brain is significantly altered immediately following mild TBI because of metabolic, hemodynamic, structural, and electrophysiologic changes. This process affects cognition and behavior and can leave the brain vulnerable for worse injury in the setting of repeat insult. This article is an update of our previously published review, reporting relevant and current studies from the bench to the bedside of mild TBI. Understanding the pathobiology can help prevent and treat mild TBI.

> Concussion associated with sport is a common occurrence with an estimated 1.6 to 3.8 million sports-related concussions yearly in the United States. The sideline assessment of concussion focuses on four areas: cognitive ability, balance, associated symptoms, and visual tracking. Tools available on the sideline to assist in the diagnosis of concussion are discussed in this article. Some of these tools are validated and reliable and some are developing and have yet to be proven to be sensitive enough for routine use. These tools along with a thorough history and physical examination enable a sideline physician to accurately diagnose concussion.

> In this review, we discuss the literature regarding concussion and mild traumatic brain injury. We focus on the role for neuroimaging in patients with suspected concussion and describe the recommended practices related to imaging in mTBI. This discussion first focuses on the exclusion of severe injuries and is followed by a discussion of the potential utility of various advanced imaging techniques in both research and clinical practice.

> Following sport-related concussion, the priorities for student athletes are return to school and extracurricular activities. Consensus-based practice

recommendations emphasize rest and gradual resumption of activities. Specific evidence-based recommendations are not available. This article provides recommendations, strategies, and a general approach to the recovery process. Most youth recover clinically and return to their normal activities within the first month following injury. It is best to avoid prolonged time off from school and restrictions on social and recreational activities because these might result in adverse consequences, such as life stress, depression, and falling behind in school.

Concussion is a physiological brain injury with physical, cognitive, and emotional sequelae. The macrophysiological insult to the brain affects the autonomic nervous system and its control of cerebral blood flow. Most patients recover within 2-4 weeks, but some do not. Persistence of symptoms beyond the generally accepted time frame for recovery is called post-concussion syndrome (PCS). PCS is not a single entity; it is a group of disorders that requires specific forms of therapy. Rest has been the mainstay of the treatment for concussion and PCS. This article discusses the rationale for the active treatment of concussion and PCS.

Persistent symptoms following concussion can be debilitating for patients and challenging for clinicians; however, evidence-based approaches to symptom management are emerging. The presentation of postconcussion syndrome can be variable among patients. Given this variability, a thorough history and physical examination are necessary to tailor an individualized treatment approach. Pharmacologic interventions can be considered when prolonged symptoms are negatively affecting quality of life. This article reviews evidence available to guide such treatment decisions.

Most people are expected to recover quickly and completely after sustaining a single, uncomplicated concussion. When unexpected difficulties are apparent or recovery is not progressing as expected, a neuropsychological evaluation may help to clarify the injury and noninjury variables that could be serving to prolong recovery. Interventions tailored to the needs of a specific patient can then be implemented to assist in improving functioning and minimizing distress.

Sport-related concussion is prevalent at all levels of play. Increased attention from sports media and scientific and medical communities has prompted players and physicians to explore the long-term effects of concussion and ask the questions of when and how players should begin to mitigate their concussion risk. The authors evaluate their risks from the perspective of epidemiology, symptomatology, neuropsychological performance, and biomechanics. The authors propose that there is not a set number of concussions that necessitates retirement in athletes and, aside from a few absolute contraindications to return to collision sport, return to play should be an individualized process.

Repeated concussive and subconcussive trauma is associated with the later development of chronic traumatic encephalopathy (CTE), a neurodegenerative disease associated with clinical symptoms in multiple domains and a unique pattern of pathologic changes. CTE has been linked to boxing and American football; CTE has also been identified in soccer, ice hockey, baseball, rugby, and military service. To date, most large studies of CTE have come from enriched cohorts associated with brain bank donations for traumatic brain injury, although several recent studies re-examining neurodegenerative disease brain banks suggest that CTE is more common than is currently appreciated.

Following the lead of Washington state and passage of the Lystedt Law in 2009, all states now have sports concussion laws designed to help protect youth athletes. This article examines the 3 basic tenets of youth sports concussion laws, challenges in implementation of state laws, and the first measures of success. Some of the major differences among state laws are also discussed.

PHYSICAL MEDICINE AND REHABILITATION CLINICS OF NORTH AMERICA

RELATED INTEREST

Neuroimaging Clinics of North America, August 2014 (Vol. 24, Issue 3)
Craniofacial Trauma
Deborah R. Shatzkes, *Editor*

VISIT THE CLINICS ONLINE!
Access your subscription at:
www.theclinics.com

Foreword

It Takes a Team Effort

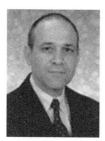

Santos F. Martinez, MD, MS
Consulting Editor

The ramifications of neurocognitive and affective sequela associated with sports and recreational-related trauma have come center stage with considerable controversy. In a society where our youth is leaning toward passive entertainment, it becomes paramount to encourage activities that promote health, fitness, and the spirit of competition. This must be balanced with safeguards and precautions to prevent injury. Many have sacrificed and been the flag bearers to bring attention to the topic of brain injury related to sports. This has been partially prompted by a number of tragedies and the unfortunate consequences that resulted in long-term challenges for the athletes and their families, which, at times, may have been prevented. Only by further research can we provide evidence-based guidance to the clinician, athlete, family, and coaches for this entity, which initially may not be so readily detectable. This will lead to further detection of high-risk demographics, patterns of play and task execution, and potential equipment shortcomings, ultimately helping identify needed regulatory changes. Screening and detection tools, neurocognitive imaging, and possibly biochemical markers may add refinement to the process. Despite our most noble efforts, however, there will be risks that must be acknowledged and vigilance must be taken by those allowing their children to participate, especially in contact sports and activities. Career athletes must become educated as to the long-term consequences of not only obvious injuries but also at times subclinically detectable trauma and their potential cumulative effects. Last, clinicians must become acquainted and up-to-date with sideline detection, management, and rehabilitation strategies to counsel and treat these athletes. The emotional inclination of banning at-risk activities must be tempered with the collaborative research and preventive efforts of clinicians, researchers, and amateur and professional sports organizations. Fortunately, such a concerted effort appears in view.

My congratulations go to Dr Laker and his fine team of contributors for making this update a great success. I would encourage clinicians caring for this population to also

Phys Med Rehabil Clin N Am 27 (2016) xi–xii
http://dx.doi.org/10.1016/j.pmr.2016.03.001
1047-9651/16/$ – see front matter © 2016 Published by Elsevier Inc.

pmr.theclinics.com

procure the February 2007 issue of *Physical Medicine and Rehabilitation Clinics of North America*, which complements this issue.

Santos F. Martinez, MD, MS
Campbell Clinic
Department of Orthopaedics
University of Tennessee
Memphis, TN, USA

E-mail address:
smartinez@campbellclinic.com

Preface

Concussion in Sports

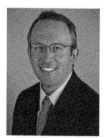

Scott R. Laker, MD
Editor

Dear colleagues,

Welcome to the issue of *Physical Medicine and Rehabilitation Clinics of North America* on concussion in sports. Few topics have seen such an increase in public awareness and medical knowledge in the last decade. We aim to update our readers on the most up-to-date information available on sports-related concussion, drawing on the original articles as a starting point for our new work from the initial concussion issue in *Physical Medicine and Rehabilitation Clinics of North America* in 2007 edited by Drs Bell and Herring.

This update gives the reader a comprehensive look at the state of the art in sport-related concussion. This issue brings the reader from pathophysiology to sideline diagnosis and management, from initial symptom management, active rehabilitation, and school interventions to the management of prolonged symptoms, and an exploration into imaging and neuropsychology, with a discussion of the impressive spread of concussion legislation, and our current understanding of chronic traumatic encephalopathy.

I would like to extend my most sincere thanks to our authors, far and wide, for their time and dedication to this issue. They are all experts in this field with decades of experience to their names. It has been a pleasure to read and be a small part of their work. I would also like to extend my personal thanks to Elsevier and Don Mumford for their strong commitment to excellence in academic writing.

I would also like to extend thanks to the athletes and families that have worked so tirelessly to make our sports world safer for youth athletes.

Personally, I would like to dedicate this issue to my friend and mentor, Dr Stanley Herring, for his career's work in the care and advocacy of youth athletes everywhere.

Yours truly,

Scott R. Laker, MD
University of Colorado School of Medicine
Aurora, CO 80045, USA

E-mail address:
SCOTT.LAKER@ucdenver.edu

Phys Med Rehabil Clin N Am 27 (2016) xiii
http://dx.doi.org/10.1016/j.pmr.2016.02.001
1047-9651/16/$ – see front matter © 2016 Published by Elsevier Inc.

pmr.theclinics.com

The Molecular Pathophysiology of Concussive Brain Injury – an Update

Garni Barkhoudarian, MD[a],*, David A. Hovda, PhD[b,c],
Christopher C. Giza, MD[d,e]

KEYWORDS

- Concussion • Traumatic brain injury • Pathophysiology • Molecular mechanisms

KEY POINTS

- Cerebral metabolism is altered immediately after concussion and may increase vulnerability for an interval after injury.
- Advanced neuroimaging, such as functional MRI, MR spectroscopy and diffusion tensor imaging can demonstrate alterations associated with concussive brain injury.
- Cumulative concussive brain injury has been associated with increased neurocognitive symtpoms.
- Pituitary dysfunction has been reported after chronic repetitive concussions and can affect quality of life.

Disclosure: These authors have nothing to disclose.
[a] Pacific Pituitary Disorders Center, John Wayne Cancer Institute, Providence Saint John's Health Center, 2200 Santa Monica Boulevard, Santa Monica, CA 90404, USA; [b] Interdepartmental Program for Neuroscience, Department of Neurosurgery, UCLA Brain Injury Research Center, Semel Institute, David Geffen School of Medicine at UCLA, Room 18-228A, 10833 Le Conte Boulevard, Los Angeles, CA 90095, USA; [c] Interdepartmental Program for Neuroscience, Department of Medical and Molecular Pharmacology, UCLA Brain Injury Research Center, Semel Institute, David Geffen School of Medicine at UCLA, Room 18-228A, 10833 Le Conte Boulevard, Los Angeles, CA 90095, USA; [d] Interdepartmental Programs for Neuroscience and Biomedical Engineering, Department of Neurosurgery, UCLA Brain Injury Research Center, Semel Institute, David Geffen School of Medicine at UCLA, Mattel Children's Hospital - UCLA, Room 18-218B, 10833 Le Conte Boulevard, Los Angeles, CA 90095, USA; [e] Interdepartmental Programs for Neuroscience and Biomedical Engineering, Division of Pediatric Neurology, Department of Pediatrics, UCLA Brain Injury Research Center, Semel Institute, David Geffen School of Medicine at UCLA, Mattel Children's Hospital - UCLA, Room 18-218B, 10833 Le Conte Boulevard, Los Angeles, CA 90095, USA
* Corresponding author.
E-mail address: barkhoudariang@jwci.org

Phys Med Rehabil Clin N Am 27 (2016) 373–393
http://dx.doi.org/10.1016/j.pmr.2016.01.003
1047-9651/16/$ – see front matter © 2016 Elsevier Inc. All rights reserved.
pmr.theclinics.com

INTRODUCTION

Concussion (mild traumatic brain injury [TBI]), particularly with organized sports, has come to the forefront of popular culture. Affecting about 1.6 million to 3.8 million athletes a year, its short-term and chronic effects have been increasingly recognized as notable sports-related injuries.[1–3] Thanks to widely disseminated checklist-based assessment tools and greater symptom awareness in the sports community, it is being diagnosed more frequently in amateur and professional venues alike. Public media have also embraced this condition, chiding collegiate coaches who ignore concussion and producing feature films depicting its chronic effects.

Nearly 20 years ago, the American Association of Neurology (AAN) introduced their grading system for the diagnosis and treatment of concussions.[4] These guidelines were focused on helping clinicians counsel patients to manage their symptoms and return to play. It has since become apparent that it is difficult to predict recovery based on initial concussion severity. The AAN released updated guidelines in 2013, based on a systematic, evidence-based review of the available literature.[5] These guidelines underscored the importance of early recognition of mild TBI to address symptoms and potentially prevent more severe injury. Early assessment tools, such as the Sports Concussion Assessment Tool, are endorsed for sideline nonphysicians with a high positive predictive value for concussion identification.[6] However, much like in consensus statements by the Concussion in Sport Group (introduced in 2001 and thrice updated),[5,7] these guidelines eliminated a severity grading system and, instead focused on factors affecting the timing of an athlete's return to play. This approach is primarily based on the presence and severity of general/neurologic symptoms or demonstrable neuropsychological impairments, as well as an individualized assessment of risk factors for prolonged recovery, such as history of prior concussions; younger age; symptoms of migraine headache, fogginess, and dizziness; learning disability or attention deficit; on-field mental status change; and possibly psychiatric comorbidities such as depression and anxiety.

Experimental animal models have been central to understanding the pathophysiology of concussive brain injury. Typically performed with rodents, techniques include closed-skull weight drop,[8,9] closed-skull controlled impact,[10,11] and lateral fluid percussion injury (FPI).[12,13] Through these models, researchers can glean clinically relevant mechanistic insight and are able to better characterize molecular alterations, ionic and neurotransmitter disturbances, synaptic perturbations, and microstructural changes. More recently, high-resolution MRI, diffusion tensor imaging (DTI)/tractography, functional MRI, and magnetic resonance (MR) spectroscopy have allowed real-time imaging of structural and molecular changes without sacrificing the animal. An added benefit is the cross-availability of these imaging modalities for human data acquisition. Such translational capacity has shown utility for bench-to-bedside research.[9,10,14–16] In particular, DTI and functional MRI have been shown to be reliable research markers of mild TBI-induced injury; identifying neuronal damage or dysfunction in the setting of otherwise normal macrostructural imaging (ie, computed tomography scanning; T1/T2 MRI).[17] Other, more invasive techniques include microdialysis of the injured brain and its histopathologic evaluation.[18,19]

This article updates our previously published article with additional focus on metabolic vulnerability to repeat injury, advanced MRI modalities assessing postconcussive outcomes, chronic changes following repetitive concussive injury, and pituitary dysfunction following prolonged exposure to mild TBI.[20]

NEUROMETABOLIC CASCADE OF CONCUSSION

The mechanical trauma exerted on the brain during a concussive event occurs via acceleration and deceleration forces on the neuronal structures. These forces set off a complex cascade of neurochemical and neurometabolic events. A mechanical disruption of cell membranes and axonal stretching causes unregulated efflux of ions through previously regulated ion channels.[21] This rapid depolarization results in indiscriminate release of numerous neurotransmitters; primarily excitatory amino acids such as glutamate.[22] This process potentiates the existing ionic flux to a wider neuronal region. Simultaneously, the Na/K ATP-dependent pump is active to reestablish ionic balance. However, this results in depleted energy stores (**Fig. 1**). These molecular cascades alone can be the cause of the postconcussive symptoms and may

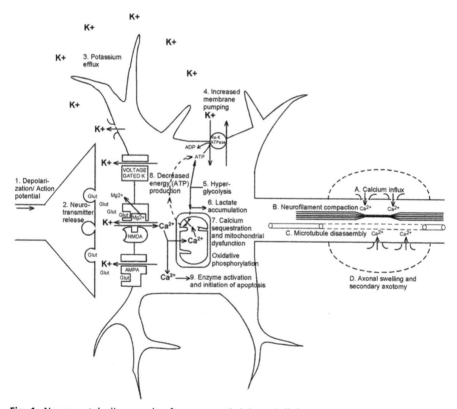

Fig. 1. Neurometabolic cascade after traumatic injury. Cellular events: (1) nonspecific depolarization and initiation of action potentials; (2) release of excitatory neurotransmitters (EAAs); (3) massive efflux of potassium; (4) increased activity of membrane ionic pumps to restore homeostasis; (5) hyperglycolysis to generate more ATP; (6) lactate accumulation; (7) calcium influx and sequestration in mitochondria, leading to impaired oxidative metabolism; (8) decreased energy (ATP) production; (9) calpain activation and initiation of apoptosis. Axonal events: (A) axolemmal disruption and calcium influx, (B) neurofilament compaction via phosphorylation or sidearm cleavage, (C) microtubule disassembly and accumulation of axonally transported organelles, (D) axonal swelling and eventual axotomy. AMPA, D-amino-3-hydroxy-5-methyl-4-isoxazolepropionic acid; Glut, glutamate; NMDA, N-methyl-D-aspartate. (*From* Giza CC, Hovda DA. The neurometabolic cascade of concussion. J Athl Train 2001;36(3):230.)

result in subsequent cerebral hypofunction or, rarely, permanent damage.[23,24] Often, these effects are self-limited and transient, although in the setting of repetitive injury this could result in more prolonged neurologic deficits. These molecular cascades are discussed in further detail later.

GLUTAMATE RELEASE AND IONIC FLUX

The deformation of neuronal membranes after biomechanical injury results in excessive potassium efflux into the extracellular space. Simultaneously, there is unregulated release of excitatory amino acids (EAAs), especially glutamate, which binds to the kainate, N-methyl D-aspartate (NMDA), and D-amino-3-hydroxy-5-methyl-4-isoxazole-propionic acid ionic channels. This process causes further regional depolarization, predominantly mediated through NMDA receptors (NMDAR); tetrodotoxin has little effect on this cascade and kynurenic acid (an NMDAR antagonist) attenuates it.[23] Hence, a widespread relative suppression of neurons occurs, creating a condition resembling spreading depression.[25–27] This concept of spreading depression has been suggested as a mechanism not only for migraine pathophysiology but also for seizures and, more recently, with secondary injury after traumatic brain injury (TBI).[28–31]

The ATP-dependent Na^+/K^+ pumps are active to maintain or normalize membrane potentials, requiring high levels of glucose metabolism, primarily through aerobic respiration. After TBI, the pump activity is maximal and quickly reduces intracellular glucose stores. As seen in experimental TBI in rats, the increased glucose metabolism occurs immediately after injury and may last from 30 minutes to 4 hours.[24] Simultaneously, there is inefficient oxidative metabolism, likely from mitochondrial dysfunction.[32,33] Hence, primarily anaerobic metabolism of glucose occurs with rampant accumulation of lactate, also seen in the extracellular space.[34] There is a resultant local acidosis, increased membrane permeability, and cerebral edema.[35] Note that lactate may be used as an energy source by neurons, once mitochondrial function resumes.[36–38] Lactate administration has been used as a treatment option for patients with severe TBI with possible positive cerebral metabolic and hemodynamic effects.[39,40]

GLUCOSE METABOLISM AND MITOCHONDRIAL EFFECTS

Following concussive injury, 2 major alterations of glucose metabolism have been described: hyperglycolysis and oxidative dysfunction. Local cerebral metabolic rates for glucose are increased within the first 30 minutes following lateral FPI, up to 30% to 46% greater than control levels.[23,24,41–43] After 6 hours, there is a relative glucose hypometabolism (approximately 50%, depending on brain region) that can last up to 5 to 10 days, depending on age, injury model, and severity. A similar profile of hyperglycolysis followed by glucose hypometabolism has been reported based on fluorodeoxyglucose (FDG)-PET measurements after human TBI. The duration of late hypometabolism may be months after moderate to severe TBI.[44] More recently, prolonged postconcussive (mild TBI) regional hypometabolism has been shown based on FDG-PET imaging compared with age-matched controls,[45,46] and has been suggested as a possible substrate of postconcussive symptoms in these patients. However, this has not yet been studied with longitudinal within-subject FDG-PET analysis.[47]

Oxidative (mitochondrial) dysfunction in the acute phase following TBI is thought to be a result of the significant influx of Ca^{++} through open NMDA channels and voltage-sensitive Ca channels. There may be resultant calcium accumulation in the mitochondria.[32,33,48,49] This calcium accumulation is reflected by decreased metabolic biomarkers such as ATP/ADP ratio, $NADH/NAD^+$ ratio, and N-acetyl aspartate

(NAA) seen after mild TBI in rat models, with lowest nadirs 3 days following injury.[9] Mitochondrial oxidative function is thought to be diminished up to 10 days following injury, partly based on downregulated cytochrome oxidase activity after FPI assessed by histochemistry.[50]

Alternative energy sources are available to the healthy and postconcussive brain. These energy sources include creatine (Cr), creatine-phosphate, and ketone bodies. Recent studies suggest that Cr and Cr-phosphate are not viable fuel sources following injury, based on decreased levels along with NAA, ATP/ADP ratio, and phosphatidyl choline following mild TBI in rats.[51] This finding was reflected in concussed athletes with decreased NAA/Cr ratios on MR spectroscopy.[52]

Ketone bodies have been known to be an alternative fuel source for the body during times of stress or starvation. Animal data suggest that although glucose metabolism is altered immediately following concussive TBI, glucose may not be the best fuel for the injured brain.[16] Ketosis or a ketogenic diet in rats following cortical contusion injury showed age-dependent decreased glucose metabolism.[16] Subsequent studies suggest that ketogenic diet is associated with smaller cerebral contusion volumes and improved behavioral outcomes.[53–55] Although the neuroprotective aspects of ketosis have yet to be systematically studied after mild TBI, it is suggested that ketosis induced by fasting may be most applicable in the first 24 hours following moderate, but not severe TBI.[56] The neuroprotective implications of ketosis have yet to be investigated systematically after mild TBI.

Repeat TBI during this period of cellular ionic disturbance, decreased cerebral blood flow, and glucose metabolic dysfunction is thought to result in more severe brain injury, described clinically as second impact syndrome.[57] However, definitive description of this clinical entity has been controversial,[7] and the role of glucose hypometabolism on brain injury has not yet been determined to be protective or exacerbating after a second insult.[58]

CEREBRAL BLOOD FLOW

Severe TBI has been associated with cerebral blood flow (CBF) perturbations, characterized by a triphasic response. This condition has been well characterized,[59] but with some variability in the degree of post-TBI ischemia.[19,60] Martin and colleagues[59] reported a series of 125 patients, assessed by cerebral arteriovenous delivery of oxygen, cerebral metabolic oxygen consumption, and vasospasm (measured by transcranial Doppler). Cerebral hypoperfusion (mean CBF, 32.3 mL/100 g/min) was noted at postinjury day (PID) 0, followed by cerebral hyperemia (mean CBF, 46.8 mL/100 g/min) and increased middle cerebral artery (MCA) velocities (86 cm/s) at PID 1 to 3. Subsequently, there is a period of cerebral vasospasm with decreased CBF of 35.7 mL/100 g/min and increased MCA velocities (96.7 cm/s)[59] at PID 4 to 15.

Decreased postinjury CBF has been shown in patients with mild TBI as well. Maugans and colleagues[61] reported a small series of pediatric patients with concussion who were evaluated with MRI CBF assessment (phase contrast quantitative flow angiography). There was a notable decrease in CBF relative to case-matched controls at initial evaluation (within 72 hours of injury: mean, 44.75 hours) of 38 ± 13.4 mL/100 g/min versus 48 ± 9.8 mL/100 g/min. Only 3 patients (27%) had recovery of CBF at 14 days, with 7 patients (67%) similarly at final follow-up (mean 41 days). There was no direct correlation with CBF rates and immediate post-concussion assessment and cognitive test (ImPACT) total symptom scores (TSS), despite increased TSS at the initial and 14-day assessments that resolved at final assessment.

These findings were supported in a recent longitudinal adult concussion athlete study by Meier and colleagues,[62] showing decreased regional CBF at 1 day and 1 week following injury relative to controls, which recovered by 1 month. There was a correlation with decreased midinsular CBF at 1 month in patients who were slower to recover. This effect has been shown in the chronic phase as well, with decreased CBF reported in symptomatic patients at 3 to 12 months following concussion.[63] The triphasic response has not been assessed in mild TBI, primarily because of the inability to reliably assess CBF data immediately after injury.

Perilesional cerebral edema assessed by MRI has been reported in animal models (cortical contusion) for severe TBI. This effect is maximal through 4 days following injury, which then recovers over the following 2 weeks correlated with the neuroscore (a behavioral scale of neurologic function).[64] Although cerebral edema was not seen in mild TBI animal models (FPI),[65] there is mild increase in the apparent diffusion coefficient with concomitant functional MRI impairment at 1 and 7 days following weight-drop injury.[15]

AXONAL INJURY AND DIFFUSION TENSOR IMAGING

In severe TBI, typically from blunt injury, diffuse axonal injury (traumatic axonal injury) has been well described. This injury is thought to be caused by the mechanical deformation of the axonal cell membranes resulting not only in the aforementioned metabolic and ionic changes[66,67] but also in neurofilament compaction. In the acute postinjury phase (5 minutes to 6 hours), this can occur by either phosphorylation or calpain-mediated proteolysis of sidearms.[68–71] Subsequently, the calcium influx can also destabilize the microtubules.[72,73] There is resultant dysfunction of axonal transport, resulting in axonal blebbing and eventual disconnection.[73–75]

This phenomenon may also occur after mild TBI, albeit with less severity and potentially reversible effects. A murine model study showed damage mainly at the axonal level, with minimal effect to the neuronal cell bodies or myelin sheaths following mild TBI via FPI.[76] This damage progressed across various cortical and subcortical structures over 4 to 6 weeks and correlated with impaired spatial learning and memory deficits (Morris water maze [MWM]). Other in vivo and in vitro models of axonal stretch show similar damage, with impaired axonal transport, axonal undulations, blebbing, and disconnection.[77]

MRI DTI and tractography are recent advances in modern imaging with significant clinical research applications. Fractional anisotropy (FA) is a measure of linear water diffusion that decreases when directionality of white matter tracts is disturbed, such as after axonal disconnection or damage to myelin sheaths[78,79] Higher FA values correlate with more linear water diffusion (ie, along tubes such as axonal tracts). Postinjury alterations in FA have been hypothesized to be related to transient axonal swelling.[80,81] This condition has been seen in pediatric, adolescent, and adult patients following mild TBI/concussion and, in some cases, has been correlated with cognitive dysfunction.[80–83]

In a pediatric study of mild and moderate TBI, FA was shown to be decreased in white matter subcortical regions (inferior frontal, superior frontal, and supracallosal), but unchanged in the corpus callosum.[84] There was a correlation of motor speed, executive function, and behavioral ratings with these FA values. Similar structural perturbations have also been seen chronically after mild TBI in adults, affecting regions such as the genu of the corpus callosum, the cingulum, the anterior corona radiata, and the uncinate fasciculus (**Fig. 2**). Although there was a direct correlation between the decrease in FA and cognitive function, there was no association with the number of

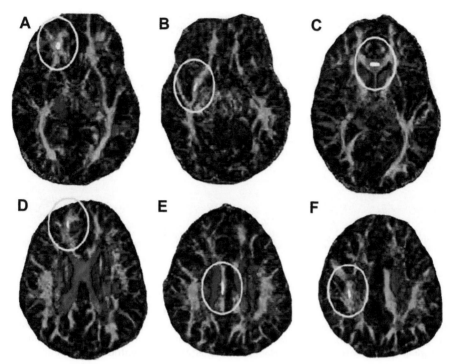

Fig. 2. Region of interest (ROI) placement for DTI. Shown are the corresponding ROIs for the right hemisphere. The solid ellipse within the yellow outlines indicates the location and size of the ROI. (*A*) Uncinate fasciculus, (*B*) inferior longitudinal fasciculus, (*C*) genu of corpus callosum, (*D*) anterior corona radiata, (*E*) cingulum bundle, and (*F*) superior longitudinal fasciculus. (*From* Niogi SN, Mukherjee P, Ghajar J, et al. Structural dissociation of attentional control and memory in adults with and without mild traumatic brain injury. Brain 2008;131:3212; with permission.)

microhemorrhages seen on high-resolution MRI. In contrast, a study in adolescent patients with mild TBI showed increased in the corpus callosum FA levels seen early (6 days) following injury (thought to be caused by axonal edema rather than disruption). However, these findings did correlate with postconcussive symptoms confirmed by cognitive, affective, and somatic scores on the Rivermead Post-Concussion Symptoms Questionnaire and Brief Symptom Inventory.[80] This increase in FA was supported by Mayer and colleagues,[85] who reported a study of 15 pediatric patients with mild TBI with increased FA scores in the corpus callosum, cingulum, internal capsule, and cerebral peduncles.

More recently, corpus callosum function has been assessed after pediatric moderate to severe TBI by interhemispheric transfer time (IHTT) using event-related potentials. There is notable variability of IHTT within sample populations, although slower IHTT has been associated with decreased performance scores.[86] Dennis and colleagues[86] reported in the slow-IHTT group a notable decrease in FA values across select axonal bundles (**Fig. 3**). In contrast, in the normal-IHTT group, there was no significant difference in FA values compared with controls. Hence, such studies support the correlation of lower FA values and impaired cognitive function via diminished connectivity.[86,87] There also seems to be a correlation with specific white matter

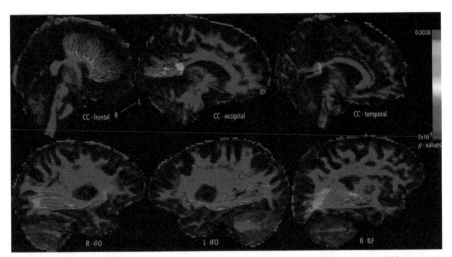

Fig. 3. Differences between IHTT-slow and control groups in FA. Whole-tract differences in FA between IHTT-slow and control. The *P* values are shown corresponding with the color bar, and results were FDR corrected across all points on all tracts tested (q < 0.05; critical *P* threshold = 0.0038). For simplicity, only tracts with at least 5% of the tract showing significant differences are displayed. CC, corpus callosum; FDR, false discovery rate; IFO, inferior fronto-occipital fasciculus; ILF, inferior longitudinal fasciculus; L, left; R, right. (*From* Dennis EL, Ellis MU, Marion SD, et al. Callosal function in pediatric traumatic brain injury linked to disrupted white matter integrity. J Neurosci 2015;35(28):10205; with permission.)

structures and select cognitive or behavioral deficits.[88] These studies suggest that DTI assessing axonal injury is a sensitive and powerful measure of the effects from TBI of all severities.

ALTERED BRAIN ACTIVATION

The NMDA glutamate receptor is of particular interest with regard to neuronal activity and calcium regulation following TBI. This tetrameric channel (2 NR1 and 2 NR2 subunits) requires 2 signals to be activated: membrane voltage change and glutamate binding. This activation releases an Mg++ ion within its working channel and allows calcium flux into the neuron. Developmentally, there is a shift of the channel composition in the rat brain, with downregulation of NR2B (slower channels) and upregulation of NR2A (faster channels) with maturity.[89]

Following lateral FPI in pediatric (postnatal day 19) rats, the relative expression of the NR2A subunit is downregulated by PID 4 with apparent recovery by PID 7.[12] The expression of NR2B and NR1 subunits remains unchanged, suggesting a possible intrinsic neuroprotective mechanism of calcium ion regulation following TBI. Long-term potentiation (LTP) and long-term depression, functions of learning and memory, are associated with NMDA channel activity and composition.[90,91] As expected, there is impaired LTP following experimental TBI, at PID 2, with apparent partial recovery by PID 7 to 15.[92,93] However, maintenance of LTP is deficient up to 8 weeks postinjury.[94]

Postconcussive patients show abnormal activation of neural circuits, associated with cognitive and behavioral deficits. Blood oxygen level–dependent sequences obtained in functional MRI before and after cognitive tasks show a hyperactivation in the postconcussive brain at 1 week (**Fig. 4**).[95,96] When abnormal activation is seen

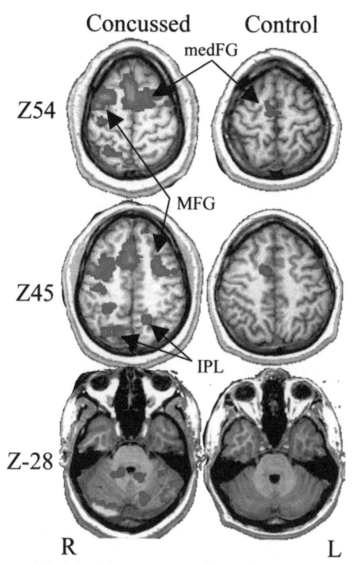

Fig. 4. Representative individual z score differences between baseline and either a postconcussion session (Concussed, *left*) or postseason baseline sessions (Control, *right*). Colored areas show regions of activity that significantly increased from the baseline value of the bimanual sequencing task. Although both concussed and control subjects show some increases in region of activity, those of the concussed players are considerably larger. Activity is significantly increased in the medial frontal gyrus (medFG), middle frontal gyrus (MFG), inferior parietal lobe (IPL), and bilateral cerebellum. (*From* Jantzen KJ, Anderson B, Steinberg FL, et al. A prospective functional MR imaging study of mild traumatic brain injury in college football players. AJNR Am J Neuroradiol 2004;25(5):741.)

following concussive brain injury, these athletes seem to have a more prolonged clinical recovery.[97,98] With task-based assessment, increased recruitment of cognitive resources has been seen, correlated with concussion severity.[96,98]

ACUTE RESPONSES TO REPEAT CONCUSSION

Although the postconcussive symptoms are important to identify and monitor, another potential reason to limit return to activity is the second impact syndrome following repeat concussive injury of the vulnerable brain.[57,99,100] Severe examples include patients with catastrophic cerebral edema following apparent mild TBI/concussion resulting in coma, severe neurologic deficits, and even death.[101–103]

Although predictive factors and the time interval for return to activity following concussion remain debated, it is evident that the cerebral physiology is altered following mild TBI, which may render the brain less functional and more vulnerable. This period of vulnerability, characterized by the aforementioned metabolic, hemodynamic, structural, and electrophysiologic dysfunction, can increase the vulnerability of the brain to repeat injury. This window of impairment has been characterized by animal studies and supported by clinical experience.[9,10,104]

A pair of recent studies attempted to assess the vulnerability interval in mice. Meehan and colleagues[105] assessed daily, weekly, and monthly repetitive concussion intervals with regard to cognitive function assessed by MWM performance. Mice sustaining 5 concussions at daily or weekly intervals had similar decreased cognitive function compared with controls. However, those sustaining 5 concussions at monthly intervals had no difference from controls. Those same mice had similar dysfunction when subsequently concussed daily. These cognitive tests suggested that concussed brain is vulnerable at up to 1 week following injury. Mannix and colleagues[106] published a follow-up long-term study showing that mice that sustained biweekly and monthly injuries did not have significant cognitive deficits. Daily and weekly concussed animals had evidence of histologic changes associated with chronic cognitive dysfunction (astrocytosis). These animal studies place the time window of vulnerability between 1 and 2 weeks following injury.

In a rat weight-drop (mild TBI) experiment by Vagnozzi and colleagues,[8] NAA, ATP, and the ATP/ADP ratio were shown to be significantly decreased at PID 2 following repeat concussion. Peak deficits were seen when repeat injuries were separated by a 3-day interval. At this combination, metabolic perturbation was similar to a single severe TBI injury. These abnormalities persisted as late as 7 days after double impact, shown in a follow-up study by the same group.[9] Adding to this, Prins and colleagues[107] assessed glucose metabolism (cerebral metabolic rate of glucose) following mild TBI in rat pups. They identified decreased glucose metabolism at PID 1 by 19%. This decrease recovered by PID 3. However, if a second injury was induced during the vulnerable period on PID 1, glucose metabolism was further depressed (36.5%) without recovery at 3 days (25% depressed metabolism). This effect was not seen when repeat injury was performed at PID 6, and correlated with working memory impairments on behavioral testing.

MR spectroscopy has proved to be a good research tool for estimating regional metabolite concentrations in athletes and other individuals with concussion.[52] In one study, 13 athletes who sustained concussions underwent 3-T MR spectroscopy at various postinjury time points. At 3 days postinjury, the NAA/Cr ratio was diminished by 18.5% compared with age-matched control patients (2.2 vs 1.8; $P<.05$). There was slight improvement at 15 days (1.88) and normalization at 30 days postinjury. Perhaps most interesting are the 3 patients who sustained a repeat concussion between 3 and

15 days after their initial injuries. These patients had a similar initial decrease in their NAA/CA ratios (1.78), but had further decrease at 15 days (1.72), rather than a partial resolution, which took 45 days to recover to baseline. The patients with single concussion reported no symptoms at the time of the 3-day study, whereas the patients with double concussion stated the same at the 30-day time point (although standardized symptom questionnaires were not administered and symptom assessments were not conducted at the intermediate time points). These findings were subsequently confirmed with a larger, multicenter cohort study of concussed athletes.[108]

Additional markers of impaired mitochondrial reductive capacity include the lactate/pyruvate ratio, which is increased in patients with severe TBI.[19,109] Therefore, it is logical to conclude that mitochondrial dysfunction increases the susceptibility for repeat injury. However, this has not been replicated in humans and MR spectroscopic data do not show statistically significant increases in the lactate ratios.[110,111]

Axonal damage is observed following mild TBI, which has been observed clinically and proved experimentally. As mentioned earlier, white matter abnormalities have been described using DTI imaging after mild TBI in humans,[80,82,112] although these findings are not universal.[113,114] Similar to the metabolic changes, this injury is also worsened by repeat concussion TBI.[11,115] This finding was shown by a repeat concussion animal model with a 3-day interval between injuries showing a significant increase in cytoskeletal damage and axonal injury.[10] A more recent murine study assessing repetitive concussion (5 concussions, 48 hours apart) not only showed worsened motor and cognitive deficits but also noted axonal injury in the corpus callosum, which was worse in the repetitive injury arm.[116] To date, there are no specific human studies of DTI conducted early after repeated concussive injuries.

Repeat mild TBI in animals acutely also induces spatial memory deficits (seen on MWM), and these impairments are related to impact severity and the number and timing of repeated injuries.[11,14,117] An National Collegiate Athletic Association (NCAA) concussion study similarly showed that athletes who sustained repeat concussions (3 or more) were at a higher risk of an additional concussion. More importantly, these patients had a significantly longer duration of postconcussive symptoms than those athletes with only 1 concussion (30% vs 14.6%).[2]

POTENTIAL FOR CUMULATIVE INJURY AND CHRONIC SEQUELAE

Patients who have sustained multiple or repetitive concussions have shown behavioral and cognitive dysfunction ranging from memory loss to gross dementia. Biological markers associated with this decline in function include amyloid and tau deposition; presence of apolipoprotein E-4 allele (ApoE-4); and overall structural damage, particularly axonal injury.

Animal studies have shown amyloid deposition in a transgenic mouse model overexpressing human amyloid precursor protein. Repetitive mild TBI resulted in significant deposition of A-β and isoprostanes, with an associated increased latency in the MWM test.[118] Others have shown increased hippocampal cell death following injury, with concomitant A-β deposition.[119,120] In contrast, some repetitive mild TBI studies have failed to show A-β deposition, although other structural deficits were noted.[106]

Chronic traumatic encephalopathy (CTE; dementia pugilistica, or punch drunkenness) has been characterized clinically since 1928.[121,122] Recently, this disorder was histopathologically characterized with deposition of tau protein, seen at autopsy in former boxers, football players, contact sport athletes, and military personnel. Immunohistochemistry shows neurofibrillary tangles and neuritic threads consistent with a generalized taupathy.[123–125] Recently, consensus pathologic criteria have been developed and agreed on at a National Institutes of Health conference (NIH).[126] Multiple animal studies also show TBI-induced abnormalities in tau and other cytoskeletal proteins.[127–130] However, the subacute time points in animal studies do not necessarily correspond to the chronic time points seen in the human neuropathological cases. McKee and colleagues[131] recently published their autopsy series of athletes and military personnel exposed to blast injury. They noted a high rate (89%) of histopathologic CTE overall in professional football athletes, although isolated CTE was noted in 63% and severe isolated CTE (stage III–IV) in 47%. Other studies have reported 32% to 87% incidence of CTE histopathology in athletes[132–134]; however, all these are selected case series from which it is not possible to extrapolate true incidence or prevalence rates.

ApoE lipoprotein and, specifically, the ApoE-4 allele are linked with development of chronic TBI.[135] This link was reported in boxers in whom a correlation was found between increased cognitive deficits, the number of boxing matches, and the ApoE-4 allele. Particularly, all patients with severe impairment as measured by the chronic brain injury scale (no tissue diagnosis) have at least 1 ApoE-4 allele.[136] Transgenic mice overexpressing ApoE-4 show more diffuse plaque formation than wild-type animals in a TBI model.[137] This finding has not yet been shown to be a factor in repetitive TBI experiments and a lack of correlation was noted by Mannix and colleagues.[106]

Axonal integrity is also degraded because of chronic repetitive TBI. DTI imaging has shown this in professional boxers with FA and whole-brain diffusion coefficients were significantly altered in boxers compared with nonboxing patients.[138] This finding has not yet been confirmed in repetitive mild TBI animal models.

In long-term studies of professional football players, there is an increased incidence of self-reported cognitive/memory deficits. In addition, there are behavioral findings, including early depression. This finding was significantly associated in players who had sustained 3 or more cumulative concussions.[139,140]

PITUITARY DYSFUNCTION

Pituitary hormonal dysfunction is known to occur in 20% to 40% of patients with moderate and severe TBI.[141–152] In these patients, hyposomatism and hypogonadism are the most common endocrinopathies, with hypothyroidism, hypocortisolism, and diabetes insipidus less common.[141–152] Certain professional athletes with repetitive mild TBI have also been shown to develop hypopituitarism with 37% to 45%or more developing at least 1 axis of pituitary dysfunction. A recent study in retired National Football League athletes showed overall hormone deficiency in 23.5% of *symptomatic* patients; primarily hyposomatism and, to a lesser extent, hypogonadism.[153] These patients also had quality-of-life metrics assessed, with a significant correlation between hormone deficiency and the International Index of Erectile Function.

Pituitary dysfunction following repetitive TBI has been replicated in animal models as well. Greco and colleagues[154] recently published their findings with repetitive brain injury in adolescent rats, with laboratory and phenotypic hyposomatism noted and direct injury to the pituitary gland seen on histopathology. Potential mechanisms of pituitary dysfunction have been proposed, including direct trauma or infarction, vascular ischemia or disruption of the portal venous system, and shear effect of the pituitary infundibulum.[155,156] Although these findings are extrapolated from data from patients with severe TBI, similar mechanisms are likely to be in effect in patients with concussion. Pituitary hormone dysfunction has been associated with decreased quality of life, and cognitive and behavioral changes, all of which can compound the illness of patients with concussion. Hormone replacement is readily available and may be considered once the hormonal dysfunction is identified.

SUMMARY

Concussion has acute and chronic detrimental effects on the brain. The cascade of molecular, hemodynamic, and electrophysiologic alterations is responsible for cognitive dysfunction and creates vulnerability for repeat injury. These effects are worsened and protracted in the setting of repeated concussions, as well as with multiple comorbidities or risk factors (migraine, learning/attention problems, younger age, anxiety/depression, etc). Pituitary hormone dysfunction can occur concomitantly, which can exacerbate these effects. Prevention and early identification of concussions should be the goal of coaches, trainers, parents, and physicians, regardless of the context of injury. Most importantly, individuals with a concussion should be protected from risk for repeat injury, which brings with it more prolonged neurobehavioral impairments and the potential for chronic or degenerative neurologic changes.

REFERENCES

1. Kelly JP, Nichols JS, Filley CM, et al. Concussion in sports. Guidelines for the prevention of catastrophic outcome. JAMA 1991;266(20):2867–9.
2. Guskiewicz KM, McCrea M, Marshall SW, et al. Cumulative effects associated with recurrent concussion in collegiate football players: the NCAA concussion study. JAMA 2003;290(19):2549–55.
3. Langlois JA, Rutland-Brown W, Wald MM. The epidemiology and impact of traumatic brain injury: a brief overview. J Head Trauma Rehabil 2006;21(5):375–8.
4. Practice parameter: the management of concussion in sports (summary statement). Report of the Quality Standards Subcommittee. Neurology 1997;48(3):581–5.
5. Giza CC, Kutcher JS, Ashwal S, et al. Summary of evidence-based guideline update: evaluation and management of concussion in sports: report of the guideline development subcommittee of the American Academy of Neurology. Neurology 2013;80(24):2250–7.
6. Barr W, McCrea M. Sensitivity and specificity of standardized neurocognitive testing immediately following sports concussion. J Int Neuropsychol Soc 2001;7(6):693.
7. McCrory P, Meeuwisse W, Johnston K, et al. Consensus statement on concussion in sport: the 3rd international conference on concussion in sport held in Zurich, November 2008. Br J Sports Med 2009;43(Suppl 1):i76–90.
8. Vagnozzi R, Signoretti S, Tavazzi B, et al. Hypothesis of the postconcussive vulnerable brain: experimental evidence of its metabolic occurrence. Neurosurgery 2005;57(1):164–71 [discussion: 164–71].
9. Vagnozzi R, Tavazzi B, Signoretti S, et al. Temporal window of metabolic brain vulnerability to concussions: mitochondrial-related impairment–part I. Neurosurgery 2007;61(2):379–88 [discussion: 388–9].
10. Longhi L, Saatman KE, Fujimoto S, et al. Temporal window of vulnerability to repetitive experimental concussive brain injury. Neurosurgery 2005;56(2):364–74 [discussion: 364–74].
11. Prins ML, Hales A, Reger ML, et al. Repeat traumatic brain injury in the juvenile rat is associated with increased axonal injury and cognitive impairments. Dev Neurosci 2010;32(4):510–8.

12. Giza CC, Maria NS, Hovda DA. N-methyl-D-aspartate receptor subunit changes after traumatic injury to the developing brain. J Neurotrauma 2006;23(6): 950–61.

13. Gurkoff GG, Giza CC, Shin D, et al. Acute neuroprotection to pilocarpine-induced seizures is not sustained after traumatic brain injury in the developing rat. Neuroscience 2009;164(2):862–76.

14. DeFord SM, Wilson MS, Rice AC, et al. Repeated mild brain injuries result in cognitive impairment in B6C3F1 mice. J Neurotrauma 2002;19(4):427–38.

15. Henninger N, Sicard KM, Li Z, et al. Differential recovery of behavioral status and brain function assessed with functional magnetic resonance imaging after mild traumatic brain injury in the rat. Crit Care Med 2007;35(11):2607–14.

16. Prins ML, Hovda DA. The effects of age and ketogenic diet on local cerebral metabolic rates of glucose after controlled cortical impact injury in rats. J Neurotrauma 2009;26(7):1083–93.

17. Difiori JP, Giza CC. New techniques in concussion imaging. Curr Sports Med Rep 2010;9(1):35–9.

18. Hillered L, Vespa PM, Hovda DA. Translational neurochemical research in acute human brain injury: the current status and potential future for cerebral microdialysis. J Neurotrauma 2005;22(1):3–41.

19. Vespa P, Bergsneider M, Hattori N, et al. Metabolic crisis without brain ischemia is common after traumatic brain injury: a combined microdialysis and positron emission tomography study. J Cereb Blood Flow Metab 2005;25(6):763–74.

20. Barkhoudarian G, Hovda D, Giza C. The molecular pathophysiology of concussive brain injury. Clin Sports Med 2011;30(1):33.

21. Farkas O, Lifshitz J, Povlishock JT. Mechanoporation induced by diffuse traumatic brain injury: an irreversible or reversible response to injury? J Neurosci 2006;26(12):3130–40.

22. Faden AI, Demediuk P, Panter SS, et al. The role of excitatory amino acids and NMDA receptors in traumatic brain injury. Science 1989;244(4906):798–800.

23. Kawamata T, Katayama Y, Hovda DA, et al. Administration of excitatory amino acid antagonists via microdialysis attenuates the increase in glucose utilization seen following concussive brain injury. J Cereb Blood Flow Metab 1992;12(1): 12–24.

24. Yoshino A, Hovda DA, Kawamata T, et al. Dynamic changes in local cerebral glucose utilization following cerebral conclusion in rats: evidence of a hyper- and subsequent hypometabolic state. Brain Res 1991;561(1):106–19.

25. Giza CC, Hovda DA. The neurometabolic cascade of concussion. J Athl Train 2001;36(3):228–35.

26. Kubota M, Nakamura T, Sunami K, et al. Changes of local cerebral glucose utilization, DC potential and extracellular potassium concentration in experimental head injury of varying severity. Neurosurg Rev 1989;12(Suppl 1):393–9.

27. Somjen GG, Giacchino JL. Potassium and calcium concentrations in interstitial fluid of hippocampal formation during paroxysmal responses. J Neurophysiol 1985;53(4):1098–108.

28. Fabricius M, Fuhr S, Willumsen L, et al. Association of seizures with cortical spreading depression and peri-infarct depolarisations in the acutely injured human brain. Clin Neurophysiol 2008;119(9):1973–84.

29. Hartings JA, Strong AJ, Fabricius M, et al. Spreading depolarizations and late secondary insults after traumatic brain injury. J Neurotrauma 2009;26(11): 1857–66.

30. Strong AJ, Fabricius M, Boutelle MG, et al. Spreading and synchronous depressions of cortical activity in acutely injured human brain. Stroke 2002;33(12):2738–43.

31. Leao AA. Further observations on the spreading depression of activity in the cerebral cortex. J Neurophysiol 1947;10(6):409–14.

32. Verweij BH, Muizelaar JP, Vinas FC, et al. Mitochondrial dysfunction after experimental and human brain injury and its possible reversal with a selective N-type calcium channel antagonist (SNX-111). Neurol Res 1997;19(3):334–9.

33. Xiong Y, Gu Q, Peterson PL, et al. Mitochondrial dysfunction and calcium perturbation induced by traumatic brain injury. J Neurotrauma 1997;14(1):23–34.

34. Kawamata T, Katayama Y, Hovda DA, et al. Lactate accumulation following concussive brain injury: the role of ionic fluxes induced by excitatory amino acids. Brain Res 1995;674(2):196–204.

35. Kalimo H, Rehncrona S, Soderfeldt B. The role of lactic acidosis in the ischemic nerve cell injury. Acta Neuropathol 1981;7:20–2.

36. Magistretti PJ, Pellerin L. Cellular mechanisms of brain energy metabolism and their relevance to functional brain imaging. Philos Trans R Soc Lond 1999;354(1387):1155–63.

37. Schurr A, Payne RS. Lactate, not pyruvate, is neuronal aerobic glycolysis end product: an in vitro electrophysiological study. Neuroscience 2007;147(3):613–9.

38. Tsacopoulos M, Magistretti PJ. Metabolic coupling between glia and neurons. J Neurosci 1996;16(3):877–85.

39. Bouzat P, Sala N, Suys T, et al. Cerebral metabolic effects of exogenous lactate supplementation on the injured human brain. Intensive Care Med 2014;40(3):412.

40. Schurr A, Gozal E. Aerobic production and utilization of lactate satisfy increased energy demands upon neuronal activation in hippocampal slices and provide neuroprotection against oxidative stress. Front Pharmacol 2011;2:96.

41. Andersen BJ, Marmarou A. Post-traumatic selective stimulation of glycolysis. Brain Res 1992;585(1–2):184–9.

42. Sunami K, Nakamura T, Ozawa Y, et al. Hypermetabolic state following experimental head injury. Neurosurg Rev 1989;12(Suppl 1):400–11.

43. Yoshino A, Hovda DA, Katayama Y, et al. Hippocampal CA3 lesion prevents postconcussive metabolic dysfunction in CA1. J Cereb Blood Flow Metab 1992;12(6):996–1006.

44. Bergsneider M, Hovda DA, Shalmon E, et al. Cerebral hyperglycolysis following severe traumatic brain injury in humans: a positron emission tomography study. J Neurosurg 1997;86(2):241–51.

45. Peskind ER, Petrie EC, Cross DJ, et al. Cerebrocerebellar hypometabolism associated with repetitive blast exposure mild traumatic brain injury in 12 Iraq war veterans with persistent post-concussive symptoms. Neuroimage 2011;54(Suppl 1):S76.

46. Provenzano F, Jordan B, Tikofsky R, et al. F-18 FDG PET imaging of chronic traumatic brain injury in boxers: a statistical parametric analysis. Nucl Med Commun 2010;31(11):952.

47. Byrnes KR, Wilson CM, Brabazon F, et al. FDG-PET imaging in mild traumatic brain injury: a critical review. Front Neuroenergetics 2013;5:13.

48. Lifshitz J, Sullivan PG, Hovda DA, et al. Mitochondrial damage and dysfunction in traumatic brain injury. Mitochondrion 2004;4(5–6):705–13.

49. Robertson CL, Saraswati M, Fiskum G. Mitochondrial dysfunction early after traumatic brain injury in immature rats. J Neurochem 2007;101(5):1248–57.

50. Hovda DA, Yoshino A, Kawamata T, et al. Diffuse prolonged depression of cerebral oxidative metabolism following concussive brain injury in the rat: a cytochrome oxidase histochemistry study. Brain Res 1991;567(1):1–10.

51. Signoretti S, Di Pietro V, Vagnozzi R, et al. Transient alterations of creatine, creatine phosphate, N-acetylaspartate and high-energy phosphates after mild traumatic brain injury in the rat. Mol Cell Biochem 2010;333(1–2):269–77.

52. Vagnozzi R, Signoretti S, Tavazzi B, et al. Temporal window of metabolic brain vulnerability to concussion: a pilot 1H-magnetic resonance spectroscopic study in concussed athletes–part III. Neurosurgery 2008;62(6):1286–95 [discussion: 1295–6].

53. Appelberg KS, Hovda DA, Prins ML. The effects of a ketogenic diet on behavioral outcome after controlled cortical impact injury in the juvenile and adult rat. J Neurotrauma 2009;26(4):497–506.

54. Arun P, Ariyannur PS, Moffett JR, et al. Metabolic acetate therapy for the treatment of traumatic brain injury. J Neurotrauma 2010;27(1):293–8.

55. Prins ML, Fujima LS, Hovda DA. Age-dependent reduction of cortical contusion volume by ketones after traumatic brain injury. J Neurosci Res 2005;82(3):413–20.

56. Davis LM, Pauly JR, Readnower RD, et al. Fasting is neuroprotective following traumatic brain injury. J Neurosci Res 2008;86(8):1812–22.

57. Cantu RC. Second-impact syndrome. Clin Sports Med 1998;17(1):37–44.

58. McCrory PR, Berkovic SF. Second impact syndrome. Neurology 1998;50(3):677–83.

59. Martin NA, Patwardhan RV, Alexander MJ, et al. Characterization of cerebral hemodynamic phases following severe head trauma: hypoperfusion, hyperemia, and vasospasm. J Neurosurg 1997;87(1):9–19.

60. Coles JP, Fryer TD, Smielewski P, et al. Incidence and mechanisms of cerebral ischemia in early clinical head injury. J Cereb Blood Flow Metab 2004;24(2):202–11.

61. Maugans TA, Farley C, Altaye M, et al. Pediatric sports-related concussion produces cerebral blood flow alterations. Pediatrics 2012;129(1):28.

62. Meier T, Bellgowan P, Singh R, et al. Recovery of cerebral blood flow following sports-related concussion. JAMA Neurol 2015;72(5):530–8.

63. Bartnik-Olson B, Holshouser B, Wang H, et al. Impaired neurovascular unit function contributes to persistent symptoms after concussion: a pilot study. J Neurotrauma 2014;31(17):1497.

64. Immonen R, Heikkinen T, Tahtivaara L, et al. Cerebral blood volume alterations in the perilesional areas in the rat brain after traumatic brain injury-comparison with behavioral outcome. J Cereb Blood Flow Metab 2010;30(7):1318–28.

65. Pasco A, Lemaire L, Franconi F, et al. Perfusional deficit and the dynamics of cerebral edemas in experimental traumatic brain injury using perfusion and diffusion-weighted magnetic resonance imaging. J Neurotrauma 2007;24(8):1321–30.

66. Mata M, Staple J, Fink DJ. Changes in intra-axonal calcium distribution following nerve crush. J Neurobiol 1986;17(5):449–67.

67. Maxwell WL, McCreath BJ, Graham DI, et al. Cytochemical evidence for redistribution of membrane pump calcium-ATPase and ecto-Ca-ATPase activity, and calcium influx in myelinated nerve fibres of the optic nerve after stretch injury. J Neurocytol 1995;24(12):925–42.

68. Johnson GV, Greenwood JA, Costello AC, et al. The regulatory role of calmodulin in the proteolysis of individual neurofilament proteins by calpain. Neurochem Res 1991;16(8):869–73.

69. Nakamura Y, Takeda M, Angelides KJ, et al. Effect of phosphorylation on 68 KDa neurofilament subunit protein assembly by the cyclic AMP dependent protein kinase in vitro. Biochem Biophys Res Commun 1990;169(2):744–50.

70. Nixon RA. The regulation of neurofilament protein dynamics by phosphorylation: clues to neurofibrillary pathobiology. Brain Pathol 1993;3(1):29–38.

71. Sternberger NH, Sternberger LA. Neurotypy: the heterogeneity of brain proteins. Ann N Y Acad Sci 1983;420:90–9.

72. Maxwell WL, Povlishock JT, Graham DL. A mechanistic analysis of nondisruptive axonal injury: a review. J Neurotrauma 1997;14(7):419–40.

73. Pettus EH, Povlishock JT. Characterization of a distinct set of intra-axonal ultrastructural changes associated with traumatically induced alteration in axolemmal permeability. Brain Res 1996;722(1–2):1–11.

74. Povlishock JT, Pettus EH. Traumatically induced axonal damage: evidence for enduring changes in axolemmal permeability with associated cytoskeletal change. Acta Neurochir Suppl 1996;66:81–6.

75. Saatman KE, Abai B, Grosvenor A, et al. Traumatic axonal injury results in biphasic calpain activation and retrograde transport impairment in mice. J Cereb Blood Flow Metab 2003;23(1):34–42.

76. Spain A, Daumas S, Lifshitz J, et al. Mild fluid percussion injury in mice produces evolving selective axonal pathology and cognitive deficits relevant to human brain injury. J Neurotrauma 2010;27(8):1429.

77. Smith DH, Johnson VE, Stewart W. Chronic neuropathologies of single and repetitive TBI: substrates of dementia? Nat Rev Neurol 2013;9(4):211–21.

78. Mac Donald CL, Dikranian K, Bayly P, et al. Diffusion tensor imaging reliably detects experimental traumatic axonal injury and indicates approximate time of injury. J Neurosci 2007;27(44):11869–76.

79. Benson RR, Meda SA, Vasudevan S, et al. Global white matter analysis of diffusion tensor images is predictive of injury severity in traumatic brain injury. J Neurotrauma 2007;24(3):446–59.

80. Wilde EA, McCauley SR, Hunter JV, et al. Diffusion tensor imaging of acute mild traumatic brain injury in adolescents. Neurology 2008;70(12):948–55.

81. Miles L, Grossman R, Johnson G, et al. Short-term DTI predictors of cognitive dysfunction in mild traumatic brain injury. Brain Inj 2008;22(2):115.

82. Niogi SN, Mukherjee P, Ghajar J, et al. Extent of microstructural white matter injury in postconcussive syndrome correlates with impaired cognitive reaction time: a 3T diffusion tensor imaging study of mild traumatic brain injury. AJNR Am J Neuroradiol 2008;29(5):967–73.

83. Lipton ML, Gellella E, Lo C, et al. Multifocal white matter ultrastructural abnormalities in mild traumatic brain injury with cognitive disability: a voxel-wise analysis of diffusion tensor imaging. J Neurotrauma 2008;25(11):1335–42.

84. Wozniak JR, Krach L, Ward E, et al. Neurocognitive and neuroimaging correlates of pediatric traumatic brain injury: a diffusion tensor imaging (DTI) study. Arch Clin Neuropsychol 2007;22(5):555–68.

85. Mayer A, Ling J, Yang Z, et al. Diffusion abnormalities in pediatric mild traumatic brain injury. J Neurosci 2012;32(50):17961.

86. Dennis EL, Ellis MU, Marion SD, et al. Callosal function in pediatric traumatic brain injury linked to disrupted white matter integrity. J Neurosci 2015;35(28):10202–11.

87. Ellis MU, Marion SD, McArthur DL, et al. The UCLA study of children with moderate-to-severe traumatic brain injury: event-related potential measure of interhemispheric transfer time. J Neurotrauma 2015. [Epub ahead of print].

88. Niogi SN, Mukherjee P, Ghajar J, et al. Structural dissociation of attentional control and memory in adults with and without mild traumatic brain injury. Brain 2008;131(Pt 12):3209–21.

89. Cull-Candy S, Brickley S, Farrant M. NMDA receptor subunits: diversity, development and disease. Curr Opin Neurobiol 2001;11(3):327–35.

90. Liu L, Wong TP, Pozza MF, et al. Role of NMDA receptor subtypes in governing the direction of hippocampal synaptic plasticity. Science 2004;304(5673):1021–4.

91. Tang YP, Wang H, Feng R, et al. Differential effects of enrichment on learning and memory function in NR2B transgenic mice. Neuropharmacology 2001;41(6):779–90.

92. Reeves TM, Lyeth BG, Povlishock JT. Long-term potentiation deficits and excitability changes following traumatic brain injury. Exp Brain Res 1995;106(2):248–56.

93. Sick TJ, Perez-Pinzon MA, Feng ZZ. Impaired expression of long-term potentiation in hippocampal slices 4 and 48 h following mild fluid-percussion brain injury in vivo. Brain Res 1998;785(2):287–92.

94. Sanders MJ, Sick TJ, Perez-Pinzon MA, et al. Chronic failure in the maintenance of long-term potentiation following fluid percussion injury in the rat. Brain Res 2000;861(1):69–76.

95. Jantzen KJ, Anderson B, Steinberg FL, et al. A prospective functional MR imaging study of mild traumatic brain injury in college football players. AJNR Am J Neuroradiol 2004;25(5):738–45.

96. Pardini J, Pardini D, Becker J, et al. Postconcussive symptoms are associated with compensatory cortical recruitment during a working memory task. Neurosurgery 2010;67(4):1020.

97. Lovell MR, Pardini JE, Welling J, et al. Functional brain abnormalities are related to clinical recovery and time to return-to-play in athletes. Neurosurgery 2007;61(2):352–9 [discussion: 359–60].

98. McAllister TW, Sparling MB, Flashman LA, et al. Neuroimaging findings in mild traumatic brain injury. J Clin Exp Neuropsychol 2001;23(6):775–91.

99. Kissick J, Johnston KM. Return to play after concussion: principles and practice. Clin J Sport Med 2005;15(6):426–31.

100. Putukian M. Repeat mild traumatic brain injury: how to adjust return to play guidelines. Curr Sports Med Rep 2006;5(1):15–22.

101. Cantu RC, Gean AD. Second-impact syndrome and a small subdural hematoma: an uncommon catastrophic result of repetitive head injury with a characteristic imaging appearance. J Neurotrauma 2010;27(9):1557.

102. Mori T, Katayama Y, Kawamata T. Acute hemispheric swelling associated with thin subdural hematomas: pathophysiology of repetitive head injury in sports. Acta Neurochir Suppl 2006;96:40.

103. McCrory P, Davis G, Makdissi M. Second impact syndrome or cerebral swelling after sporting head injury. Curr Sports Med Rep 2012;11(1):21.

104. Tavazzi B, Vagnozzi R, Signoretti S, et al. Temporal window of metabolic brain vulnerability to concussions: oxidative and nitrosative stresses–part II. Neurosurgery 2007;61(2):390–5 [discussion: 395–6].

105. Meehan W 3rd, Zhang J, Mannix R, et al. Increasing recovery time between injuries improves cognitive outcome after repetitive mild concussive brain injuries in mice. Neurosurgery 2012;71(4):885.
106. Mannix R, Meehan W, Mandeville J, et al. Clinical correlates in an experimental model of repetitive mild brain injury. Ann Neurol 2013;74(1):65.
107. Prins ML, Alexander D, Giza CC, et al. Repeated mild traumatic brain injury: mechanisms of cerebral vulnerability. J Neurotrauma 2013;30(1):30.
108. Vagnozzi R, Signoretti S, Cristofori L, et al. Assessment of metabolic brain damage and recovery following mild traumatic brain injury: a multicentre, proton magnetic resonance spectroscopic study in concussed patients. Brain 2010; 133(11):3232.
109. Vespa P, Boonyaputthikul R, McArthur DL, et al. Intensive insulin therapy reduces microdialysis glucose values without altering glucose utilization or improving the lactate/pyruvate ratio after traumatic brain injury. Crit Care Med 2006;34(3):850–6.
110. Tremblay S, Beaulé V, Proulx S, et al. Multimodal assessment of primary motor cortex integrity following sport concussion in asymptomatic athletes. Clin Neurophysiol 2014;125(7):1371.
111. Gardner A, Iverson G, Stanwell P. A systematic review of proton magnetic resonance spectroscopy findings in sport-related concussion. J Neurotrauma 2014; 31(1):1.
112. Huang MX, Theilmann RJ, Robb A, et al. Integrated imaging approach with MEG and DTI to detect mild traumatic brain injury in military and civilian patients. J Neurotrauma 2009;26(8):1213–26.
113. Levin HS, Wilde E, Troyanskaya M, et al. Diffusion tensor imaging of mild to moderate blast-related traumatic brain injury and its sequelae. J neurotrauma 2010; 27(4):683–94.
114. Schrader H, Mickeviciene D, Gleizniene R, et al. Magnetic resonance imaging after most common form of concussion. BMC Med Imaging 2009;9:11.
115. Laurer HL, Bareyre FM, Lee VM, et al. Mild head injury increasing the brain's vulnerability to a second concussive impact. J Neurosurg 2001;95(5):859–70.
116. Mouzon B, Chaytow H, Crynen G, et al. Repetitive mild traumatic brain injury in a mouse model produces learning and memory deficits accompanied by histological changes. J Neurotrauma 2012;29(18):2761.
117. DeRoss AL, Adams JE, Vane DW, et al. Multiple head injuries in rats: effects on behavior. J Trauma 2002;52(4):708–14.
118. Uryu K, Laurer H, McIntosh T, et al. Repetitive mild brain trauma accelerates Aβ deposition, lipid peroxidation, and cognitive impairment in a transgenic mouse model of Alzheimer amyloidosis. J Neurosci 2002;22(2):446–54.
119. Rabadi MH, Jordan BD. The cumulative effect of repetitive concussion in sports. Clin J Sport Med 2001;11(3):194–8.
120. Smith DH, Nakamura M, McIntosh TK, et al. Brain trauma induces massive hippocampal neuron death linked to a surge in beta-amyloid levels in mice overexpressing mutant amyloid precursor protein. Am J Pathol 1998;153(3):1005–10.
121. Critchley M. Medical aspects of boxing, particularly from a neurological standpoint. Br Med J 1957;1(5015):357.
122. Martland, Harrison S. Punch drunk. JAMA 1928;91:1103–7.
123. McKee AC, Cantu RC, Nowinski CJ, et al. Chronic traumatic encephalopathy in athletes: progressive tauopathy after repetitive head injury. J Neuropathol Exp Neurol 2009;68(7):709–35.

124. Omalu BI, Hamilton RL, Kamboh MI, et al. Chronic traumatic encephalopathy (CTE) in a National Football League player: case report and emerging medico-legal practice questions. J Forensic Nurs 2010;6(1):40–6.

125. Smith C, Graham DI, Murray LS, et al. Tau immunohistochemistry in acute brain injury. Neuropathol Appl Neurobiol 2003;29(5):496–502.

126. McKee AC, Cairns NJ, Dickson DW, et al. The first NINDS/NIBIB consensus meeting to define neuropathological criteria for the diagnosis of chronic traumatic encephalopathy. Acta Neuropathol 2016;131(1):75–86.

127. Genis L, Chen Y, Shohami E, et al. Tau hyperphosphorylation in apolipoprotein E-deficient and control mice after closed head injury. J Neurosci Res 2000; 60(4):559–64.

128. Hoshino S, Tamaoka A, Takahashi M, et al. Emergence of immunoreactivities for phosphorylated tau and amyloid-beta protein in chronic stage of fluid percussion injury in rat brain. Neuroreport 1998;9(8):1879–83.

129. Kanayama G, Takeda M, Niigawa H, et al. The effects of repetitive mild brain injury on cytoskeletal protein and behavior. Methods Find Exp Clin Pharmacol 1996;18(2):105–15.

130. Smith DH, Chen XH, Nonaka M, et al. Accumulation of amyloid beta and tau and the formation of neurofilament inclusions following diffuse brain injury in the pig. J Neuropathol Exp Neurol 1999;58(9):982–92.

131. McKee AC, Stein TD, Nowinski CJ, et al. The spectrum of disease in chronic traumatic encephalopathy. Brain 2013;136(1):43.

132. Omalu B, Bailes J, Hamilton R, et al. Emerging histomorphologic phenotypes of chronic traumatic encephalopathy in American athletes. Neurosurgery 2011; 69(1):173.

133. Hazrati L-N, Tartaglia MC, Diamandis P, et al. Absence of chronic traumatic encephalopathy in retired football players with multiple concussions and neurological symptomatology. Front Hum Neurosci 2013;7:222.

134. Bieniek KF, Ross OA, Cormier KA, et al. Chronic traumatic encephalopathy pathology in a neurodegenerative disorders brain bank. Acta Neuropathol 2015; 130(6):877–89.

135. Jordan BD. Chronic traumatic brain injury associated with boxing. Semin Neurol 2000;20(2):179–85.

136. Jordan BD, Relkin NR, Ravdin LD, et al. Apolipoprotein E epsilon4 associated with chronic traumatic brain injury in boxing. JAMA 1997;278(2):136–40.

137. Hartman RE, Laurer H, Longhi L, et al. Apolipoprotein E4 influences amyloid deposition but not cell loss after traumatic brain injury in a mouse model of Alzheimer's disease. J Neurosci 2002;22(23):10083–7.

138. Zhang L, Heier LA, Zimmerman RD, et al. Diffusion anisotropy changes in the brains of professional boxers. AJNR Am J Neuroradiol 2006;27(9):2000–4.

139. Guskiewicz KM, Marshall SW, Bailes J, et al. Association between recurrent concussion and late-life cognitive impairment in retired professional football players. Neurosurgery 2005;57(4):719–26 [discussion: 719–26].

140. Guskiewicz KM, Marshall SW, Bailes J, et al. Recurrent concussion and risk of depression in retired professional football players. Med Sci Sports Exerc 2007;39(6):903–9.

141. Agha A, Rogers B, Sherlock M, et al. Anterior pituitary dysfunction in survivors of traumatic brain injury. J Clin Endocrinol Metab 2004;89(10):4929–36.

142. Aimaretti G, Ambrosio MR, Di Somma C, et al. Traumatic brain injury and subarachnoid haemorrhage are conditions at high risk for hypopituitarism: screening study at 3 months after the brain injury. Clin Endocrinol 2004;61(3):320–6.

143. Aimaretti G, Ambrosio MR, Di Somma C, et al. Residual pituitary function after brain injury-induced hypopituitarism: a prospective 12-month study. J Clin Endocrinol Metab 2005;90(11):6085–92.
144. Bondanelli M, De Marinis L, Ambrosio MR, et al. Occurrence of pituitary dysfunction following traumatic brain injury. J Neurotrauma 2004;21(6):685–96.
145. Herrmann BL, Rehder J, Kahlke S, et al. Hypopituitarism following severe traumatic brain injury. Exp Clin Endocrinol Diabetes 2006;114(6):316–21.
146. Kelly DF, Gonzalo IT, Cohan P, et al. Hypopituitarism following traumatic brain injury and aneurysmal subarachnoid hemorrhage: a preliminary report. J Neurosurg 2000;93(5):743–52.
147. Leal-Cerro A, Flores JM, Rincon M, et al. Prevalence of hypopituitarism and growth hormone deficiency in adults long-term after severe traumatic brain injury. Clin Endocrinol 2005;62(5):525–32.
148. Lieberman SA, Oberoi AL, Gilkison CR, et al. Prevalence of neuroendocrine dysfunction in patients recovering from traumatic brain injury. J Clin Endocrinol Metab 2001;86(6):2752–6.
149. Tanriverdi F, Senyurek H, Unluhizarci K, et al. High risk of hypopituitarism after traumatic brain injury: a prospective investigation of anterior pituitary function in the acute phase and 12 months after trauma. J Clin Endocrinol Metab 2006;91(6):2105–11.
150. Ware J Jr, Sherbourne C, The MOS. 36-item short-form health survey (SF-36). I. Conceptual framework and item selection. Med Care 1992;30(6):473.
151. Ware JE, Kosinski M. SF-36 physical & mental health summary scales: a manual for users of version 1. Lincoln (RI): Quality Metric; 2001.
152. Bavisetty S, McArthur D, Dusick J, et al. Chronic hypopituitarism after traumatic brain injury: risk assessment and relationship to outcome. Neurosurgery 2008; 62(5):1080.
153. Kelly D, Chaloner C, Evans D, et al. Prevalence of pituitary hormone dysfunction, metabolic syndrome, and impaired quality of life in retired professional football players: a prospective study. J Neurotrauma 2014;31(13):1161.
154. Greco T, Hovda D, Prins M. The effects of repeat traumatic brain injury on the pituitary in adolescent rats. J Neurotrauma 2013;30(23):1983.
155. Kornblum R, Fisher R. Pituitary lesions in craniocerebral injuries. Arch Pathol 1969;88(3):242.
156. Ceballos R. Pituitary changes in head trauma (analysis of 102 consecutive cases of head injury). Ala J Med Sci 1966;3(2):185.

Sideline Management of Concussion

 CrossMark

John Hyden, MD[a,b,*], Benjamin Petty, MD[a,b]

KEYWORDS

- Sideline • Concussion • SCAT3 • Balance • Vision • Symptom scale

KEY POINTS

- Concussion is a common occurrence in the athletic setting, and can be difficult to diagnose in a sideline situation.
- History and physical examination are important aspects of the evaluation of potential concussion with an emphasis placed on associated symptoms and a complete neurologic examination.
- The SCAT3 is a vital and important test that can be used on the sidelines to evaluate a potential concussion.
- There are other sideline tools to measure vision, reaction time, neurocognitive processes, and head impact/acceleration that are used in the sideline evaluation of concussion.
- An ideal sideline concussion evaluation test should be quick, cost effective, easy to administer, and reproducible.

INTRODUCTION

Concussion is defined as a complex pathophysiologic process affecting the brain caused by biomechanical forces. These forces can either be direct (eg, the head, neck, or face striking another object) or indirect (eg, impulsive forces transmitted to the head from a force somewhere else on the body).[1] It is estimated that there are 1.6 to 3.8 million sports-related concussions in the United States on an annual basis.[2] There is evidence that children (ages 5–18) may be more susceptible to concussion and can take longer to recover.[3] It is also known that athletes who have experienced multiple concussions in the past may be more susceptible to future concussions, suffer subsequent concussions with less force, and potentially take longer to recover.[4] Females may be more susceptible, and there may also be genetic traits[5] that increase the risk of sustaining a concussion.[3,6] Concussion rate varies by the sport with American football (3.02 per 1000 athlete exposures), ice hockey (1.96 per 1000 athlete

Disclosure Statement: The authors have nothing to disclose.
[a] Campbell Clinic Orthopaedics, 1400 South Germantown Road, Germantown, TN 38138, USA;
[b] University of Tennessee Health Science Center, Memphis, TN, USA
* Corresponding author. 1400 South Germantown Road, Germantown, TN 38138.
E-mail address: jhyden@campbellclinic.com

exposures), and women's soccer (1.80 per 1000 athlete exposures) being the most prevalent sports.[7]

The onset of symptoms is rapid or delayed, making the diagnosis of concussion difficult in the acute setting. In addition, athletes may hide symptoms to continue playing. McCrea and coworkers[8] in 2004 published a study that showed that 50% to 75% of sports concussions go unreported at the high school level. A study done in 2013 at the University of Pennsylvania by Torres and colleagues[9] indicated that 43% of athletes had knowingly hidden a concussion from their athletic trainer or coach and 22% of athletes would be likely to hide a concussion again if the situation arose. The long-term and delayed effects of concussion are still a developing and controversial subject. However, there is evidence that exposure to repeated concussions can lead to prolonged symptoms, and may increase the risk of developing psychiatric illnesses, dementia, and chronic traumatic encephalopathy.[10] The clinical diagnosis of concussion is based on a variety of factors combined with a high degree of suspicion. There is no completely reliable sideline test that can replace clinical judgment. The sideline assessment of concussion is challenging at times; however, there are tools available to help in this process.

PHYSICAL EXAMINATION

After an athlete is suspected of suffering a concussion, the athlete should be held out of participation until assessed by a licensed health care professional. In an ideal situation, the team physician or athletic trainer, who are specifically trained in concussion diagnosis and management, would be present to assess and manage the injury. It is understood that there are many instances in which there is not an athletic trainer or physician on the sidelines, making it important for coaches and parents to be educated on the signs and symptoms of concussion. If there is concern for concussion, the athlete should not return to play and should be assessed by a health care professional as soon as possible.[1] There are some signs/or symptoms that could warrant emergent transfer to a hospital including the following:

- Prolonged loss of consciousness
- Multiple episodes of vomiting
- Progressive worsening of symptoms
- Signs of a potential skull fracture
- Focal findings on neurologic examination
- Decreasing level of consciousness

If any of these symptoms are present, the emergency action system should be activated and the athlete should be transferred to the nearest hospital.

The initial part of the examination should focus on the potential injury to the cervical spine. If an athlete loses consciousness then a cervical spine injury should be assumed until ruled out. The cervical spine should be immobilized on the field and an immediate spine and neurologic examination should take place. If a cervical spine injury is suspected then the athlete should be transferred emergently via ambulance using a spine board for immobilization to the nearest hospital for further assessment and management. After ruling out a significant cervical spine injury on the sideline, neurologic examination should include the following:

- Cranial nerve function testing
- Upper and lower extremity neurologic examination with emphasis on sensation, reflexes, and strength

- Balance assessment
- Coordination assessment
- Evaluation of cognitive processing

The athlete should be monitored serially for worsening or change in symptoms. It is important that the athlete not be left alone at any time during this process. If available, an athletic trainer or team physician should stay with the athlete, although a parent, adult, or student may be used if necessary. If there is concern for worsening or a change in signs or symptoms then the athlete should be examined thoroughly again and appropriate measures should be taken. Serial evaluations every 30 minutes should take place until the athlete stabilizes or is transported to another health care facility. It is also appropriate to send the athlete home with instructions on care for concussion and the signs and symptoms to monitor.[3] Many states require this type of notification to be provided to parents. Providers should review their state and local policy regarding parental notification. An example of these instructions is included next.

Watch for Any of the Following Problems

- Difficulty remembering recent events
- Slurring of speech
- Worsening headache
- Stumbling/loss of balance
- Vomiting
- Weakness in one arm/leg
- Decreased level of consciousness
- Blurred vision
- Dilated pupils
- Confusion
- Increased irritability
- Ringing in ears

An Example of Take Home Instructions

It is okay to use acetaminophen for headache or pain, use an ice pack for comfort, eat a light meal, and go to sleep. There is no need to check eyes with a light, wake up every hour, or stay in bed. Do not drink alcohol; drive a car; or use aspirin, ibuprofen, or other nonsteroidal anti-inflammatory drug products.

Under no circumstance should an athlete suspected of sustaining a concussion be allowed to return to play without being cleared by a health care professional. With that being said, precautions should be taken by those who care for athletes, and it is never wrong to withhold an athlete from competition if there is any question as to whether a concussion has occurred. No athlete should be allowed to return to play on the same day as sustaining a concussion, and there are now clear evidence-based guidelines about return to play that are supported by state law in every state. Health care professionals do have some validated and some unvalidated tools that could potentially aid in the sideline assessment of concussion, but these tools should not replace the importance of high clinical suspicion in the diagnosis of concussion.

SYMPTOM CHECKLIST

The simplest and quickest way to assess for concussion is to do a symptom checklist. Also called a postconcussion symptom scale, this checklist contains common signs and symptoms that are associated with concussion. It consists of items that are scored on a seven-point Likert scale (0–6) with zero being asymptomatic and six being very symptomatic.[11]

Symptoms associated with concussion can manifest in many different ways. Some of these symptoms are present on the sidelines and some both on the sidelines and in follow-up.[12]

Somatic

- Headache
- Dizziness
- Balance disruption
- Nausea/vomiting
- Photophobia
- Phonophobia
- Blurry vision

Cognitive

- Confusion
- Anterograde amnesia
- Retrograde amnesia
- Loss of consciousness
- Disorientation
- Feeling mentally "foggy"
- Inability to focus
- Delayed verbal and motor responses
- Slurred/incoherent speech
- Excessive drowsiness

Affective

- Emotional lability
- Irritability
- Fatigue
- Anxiety
- Sadness

Sleep

- Trouble falling asleep
- Sleeping more than usual
- Sleeping less than usual

The first team to use this as an evaluation tool was the Pittsburgh Steelers of the National Football League.[13] Since they adopted this symptom checklist approach multiple professional, colleges, and high schools across the country also have used it. The checklist can also be used to assess the progression of symptoms over a short or prolonged period of time, and can be used to determine when return to play can commence. The number of items on the checklist varies from 22 on the sport concussion assessment tool (SCAT), the Steelers version containing 17 items, and another common version called the concussion symptom inventory containing only 12 items. The presence of symptoms associated with concussion cannot diagnose a concussion but can lead to further evaluation or precautions before making return to play decisions.

MADDOCKS QUESTIONS

The Maddocks questions have become a main component of sideline assessment of concussion and are included in the SCAT3 and standardized assessment of concussion (SAC,) which are widely used today. Maddocks and coworkers[14] developed the questions to assess the sensitivity of orientation and recent memory in the diagnosis of concussion. The results show that items evaluating recently acquired information are more sensitive in the assessment of concussion than standard orientation items. The five questions focus on short- and intermediate-term memory and can be used on the sidelines of a game. The questions are as follows:

- Where are we?
- What quarter/half is it right now?
- Who scored last in the game/practice?
- Who did we play in the last game?
- Did we win the last game?

One point is given for each correct answer and zero points are given for each incorrect or incoherent answer. This is a simple tool that can be used by health care professionals, coaches, and parents that can help in the diagnosis of concussion and should be repeated serially every 30 minutes on the sidelines.[14]

STANDARDIZED ASSESSMENT OF CONCUSSION

The SAC is a tool that has been developed to assess orientation, immediate memory, concentration, and delayed recall in an athletic setting.[15] **Fig. 1** shows a sample

Orientation: (1 point each)
Month
Date
Day of week
Year
Time (within 1 hr)
Orientation score: 5

Immediate Memory: (1 point for each correct, total over 3 trials)

	Trial 1	Trial 2	Trial 3
Word 1			
Word 2			
Word 3			
Word 4			
Word 5			

Immediate Memory score: 15

Concentration:
Reverse digits. (Go to next string length if correct on first trial. Stop if incorrect on both trials. 1 point each for each string length.)

3-8-2	5-1-8
2-7-9-3	2-1-6-8
5-1-8-6-9	9-4-1-7-5
6-9-7-3-5-1	4-2-8-9-3-7

Months of the year in reverse order. (1 point for entire sequence correct.)
Dec-Nov-Oct-Sep-Aug-Jul
Jun-May-Apr-Mar-Feb-Jan
Concentration score: 5

Delayed Recall: (approximately 5 minutes after Immediate Memory. 1 point each.)
Word 1
Word 2
Word 3
Word 4
Word 5
Delayed Recall score: 5

Summary of total scores

Orientation	5
Immediate Memory	15
Concentration	5
Delayed Recall	5
Total score	30

The following may be performed between the Immediate Memory and Delayed Recall portions of this assessment when appropriate:

Neurologic Screening:
Recollection of the injury:
Strength:
Sensation:
Coordination:

Exertional Maneuvers:
1 40-yard sprint
5 sit-ups
5 push-ups
5 knee bends

Fig. 1. Standardization assessment of concussion. (*From* McCrea M, Kelly JP, Kluge J, et al. Standardized assessment of concussion in football players. Neurology 1997;48(3):587; with permission.)

of the SAC.[16] The SAC is separated into four sections. The first section tests orientation and is similar to the Maddocks questions. It consists of the following questions:

- What month is it?
- What is the date?
- What day of the week is it?
- What year is it?
- What time is it (within 1 hour)?

One point is given for each correct answer and zero points for each incorrect answer with a total possible score of five points.

The second section tests immediate memory and consists of five simple words that are repeated three times. The person administering this section says the five words and the athlete repeats them. This process is repeated for a total of three times. One point is given for each correct answer and a zero is given for each incorrect answer with a total possible score of 15.

The third section assesses concentration. The examiner begins with a string of three numbers and the athlete repeats them back in reverse order. The athlete has two chances to get it correct, and if correct then four numbers, five numbers, and up to six numbers are attempted until there are two incorrect answers in a row. One point is given for each correct answer with a maximum possible score of four. The athlete is then asked to list the months of the year in reverse order starting with December. A score of one is given if the athlete is able to list all of the months correctly. In this section there is a maximum possible score of five points.

The fourth section tests delayed recall and asks the athlete to repeat the five words that were given in the second section. This is done at the end of the other sections to ensure that it is done in a delayed manner. One point is given for each correct word with a total possible score of five points. The scores from each section are totaled with a total possible score of 30 points.

McCrea[15] studied the efficacy of the SAC in detecting abnormalities that result from concussion in high school and college athletes. A baseline SAC was obtained in the preseason and the SAC was repeated immediately after the athlete was diagnosed with a concussion. The athletes diagnosed with a concussion on average scored four points below their baseline score. A control group of athletes showed no decrease from baseline. A score of one below baseline was 95% sensitive and 76% specific in identifying those athletes who sustained a concussion. Other studies have questioned the validity of the SAC because it may be too easy and lack acceptable discrimination to have a reliable baseline.[17]

BALANCE ERROR SCORING SYSTEM

The balance error scoring system (BESS) was developed by Guskiewicz and colleagues[18] at the University of North Carolina in 2001. Balance is integral to daily activities and sport and involves multiple neurologic systems including the vestibular, visual, and somatosensory. The theory behind the BESS is that balance is altered when an athlete suffers a concussion. The test includes three stances (**Fig. 2**)[19]: (1) double leg (hands on the hips and feet together), (2) single-leg stance (standing on nondominant leg with hands on hips), and (3) tandem stance (nondominant foot behind dominant foot, heel to toe).

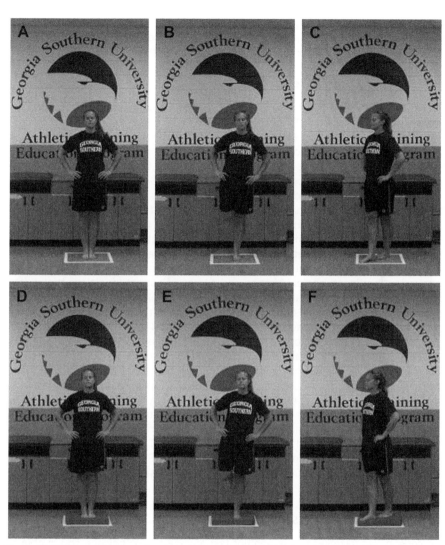

Fig. 2. (*A–F*) Balance error scoring system. (*From* Burk JM, Munkasy BA, Joyner AB, et al. Balance error scoring system performance changes after a competitive athletic season. Clin J Sport Med 2013;23(4):314; with permission.)

Each stance is done on a hard, flat surface for 20 seconds with the eyes closed. An error is defined as opening eyes, lifting hands off hips, stepping, stumbling or falling out of position, lifting forefoot or heel, abducting the hip by more than 30°, or failing to return to the test position in more than 5 seconds. The maximum number of errors that is recorded for each stance is 10, with a total maximum score of 30. If available, it is important to compare with the baseline. Multiple studies have been developed trying assess the reliability and sensitivity of the BESS in the diagnosis of concussion. Bell and coworkers[20] performed a systematic review in 2011 and found that athletes who have experienced a concussion average 17 errors compared with a baseline average of 10 errors. Scores tend to increase with concussion, postural ankle instability, external ankle taping, fatigue, and age.[20]

There are other means of measuring balance that are being used but may not be as easy to use on the sidelines including force plate balance testing and Wii fit balance testing. The BESS is incorporated in a modified way on the SCAT3.

SPORT CONCUSSION ASSESSMENT TOOL

The SCAT is now in its third version (SCAT3) and was released after the fourth International Conference on Concussion in Sport in Zurich in 2013.[1] A free copy is available online through the *British Journal of Sports Medicine* designed for health care professionals and a pocket version is available for nonprofessionals. This tool combines the following tools: Maddocks questions, the SAC, a modified BESS, the Glasgow Coma Scale, and coordination testing. The SCAT3 begins with a description of the test itself and its potential utility. Next it gives a definition of concussion, indications for emergency management, and a listing of potential signs of concussion. This is followed by the Glasgow Coma Scale, Maddocks questions, and description of the mechanism of the injury. The next section includes a background description of the athlete that includes name, age, gender, number of previous concussions, date of last concussion, amount of time required to recover from last concussion, pertinent medical history, and names of current medicines the athlete is taking. The symptom evaluation checklist is next followed by a modified SAC without the orientation questions. A neck examination is then performed with a focus on range of motion, tenderness, and upper and lower extremity sensation and strength. The final part of the SCAT3 uses a modified BESS (ie, the testing occurs only on a firm surface) and a coordination test that consists of a finger-to-nose task. Also included are specific instructions for the test, signs to look out for in the immediate time after a concussion, a suggestion on how to return to play, concussion injury advice, and a scoring summary. Although not necessary, having a baseline SCAT3 is useful in assessing the potential effects of a concussion on the athlete. This test is recommended for athletes 13 years of age or older. There is a child SCAT3 for athletes 12 and younger.[1] The SCAT3 was developed because there were questions surrounding the sensitivity of the SCAT2.[21] At this point there are no definitive studies that validate the use of the SCAT3 as a definitive tool in the diagnosis of concussion.[22]

SENSORY ORGANIZATION TEST

The sensory organization test is another test that measures balance and is able to evaluate the vestibular, visual, and somatosensory systems. A visual example of the sensory organization test is shown in **Fig. 3**.[23] Each of these three systems are evaluated with eyes open and closed on a fixed force plate and a calibrated sway reference force plate giving six different conditions tested. The purpose of this test is to assess the athlete's ability to maintain postural ability and balance with or without vision and with or without movement. After the test is performed a report is produced that measures the following:

- Center of gravity
- Ability to incorporate somatosensory input into balance
- Ability to incorporate visual input into balance
- Ability to incorporate vestibular input into balance
- Preference: how much the athlete relies on vision for balance
- Compensation assessment: does the athlete rely primarily on ankle or hip for balance

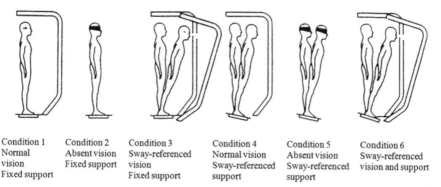

Condition 1	Condition 2	Condition 3	Condition 4	Condition 5	Condition 6
Normal vision	Absent vision	Sway-referenced vision	Normal vision	Absent vision	Sway-referenced vision and support
Fixed support	Fixed support	Fixed support	Sway-referenced support	Sway-referenced support	

Fig. 3. Sensory organization test. (*From* Yeh JR, Hsu LC, Lin C, et al. Nonlinear analysis of sensory organization test for subjects with unilateral vestibular dysfunction. PLoS One 2014;9(3):e91230; with permission.)

This test may be capable of finding subtle changes in balance that simpler tests, such as the BESS, are unable to measure.[24] This test may also be more sensitive than the BESS in diagnosing balance difficulties associated with a potential concussion.[24] The cost and relative difficulty with applying it on the sidelines make this test less applicable in a game situation.

KING-DEVICK

Concussion can commonly affect the visual pathways. There are sideline tests that assess cognition and balance, but these do not include an assessment of vision. King-Devick is a vision test that uses rapid number reading of three cards with variably spaced single digits. **Fig. 4**[25] provides an example of the King-Devick cards. The athlete is instructed to read the numbers on each card from left to right as quickly as possible. The time it takes to read each card is recorded and summed up to get a total time score. The test generally takes less than 2 minutes to administer. The King-Devick test has been used in multiple athletic settings and is easily used by nonmedical personnel, such as parents or coaches. Multiple studies have shown that King-Devick times worsen (increase) in athletes who have a concussion when compared with baseline.[26] Studies have also shown that time scores improve (decrease) with fatigue, repeat testing, and increased age.[26] There is no specific change in score from baseline that can determine whether or not an athlete has sustained a concussion; however, any worsening or slowing of the time score from baseline should raise concern. This test is a simple, rapid, objective tool that is low cost and is used easily on the sidelines.

REACTION TIME

Prolonged reaction time is a common symptom associated with sports-related concussion. A simple test to measure reaction time has been developed at the University of Michigan by Eckner and colleagues[27] and can be used to help in the diagnosis of concussion. An 80-cm long stick with a weighted rubber disk (hockey puck) is used for this test. Athletes sit with their dominant arm resting on the edge of a table with their hand surrounding but not touching the weighted rubber disk. The stick is held by the examiner with the top face of the disk aligned with the top of the athlete's hand. After random delays ranging from 2 to 5 seconds the examiner drops the stick and the

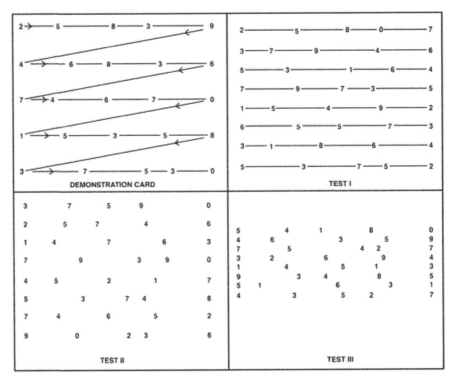

Fig. 4. King-Devick cards. (*From* Galetta KM, Morganroth J, Moehringer N, et al. Adding vision to concussion testing: a prospective study of sideline testing in youth and collegiate athletes. J Neuroophthalmol 2015;35(3):235–41.)

athlete catches it as quickly as possible by closing his or her hand. There are two practice trials followed by eight data acquisition trials. A reaction time is obtained for each trial from the distance traveled by the device using the formula for body falling under the influence of gravity. The mean value of the eight trials is obtained compared with baseline and a change score is determined. A positive change score indicates a worsening from baseline and a negative change score indicates an improvement. Additional studies of the drop stick test have shown that it is valid and reliable for college athletes, seems to be sensitive to the effects of concussion, can effectively distinguish the concussed from the nonconcussed athlete, and correlates with reaction time measured with computer-based neurocognitive testing.[28] Given its simplicity, low cost, and the small amount of time it takes to administer this test it is a viable option in sideline assessment of concussion.

ELECTROENCEPHALOGRAPHY

Electroencephalography (EEG) is a tool commonly used to assess cerebral function following a traumatic brain injury. Although not commonly used as a sideline assessment for concussion, the ease of portability could allow it to be a useable tool in the sports setting. A digital recording of the functioning of the brain is acquired from 21 electrodes attached to the scalp and waveforms are generated and interpreted. Analysis of the data can show abnormal brain patterns that are known to be consistent with concussion. Abnormal findings can include generalized or focal slowing and attenuated posterior alpha. The severity and duration of these abnormal findings tend to vary with injury severity. Typically the more severe the concussion, the more likely there are abnormalities on EEG. There are also many other comorbidities that could show similar abnormalities on EEG including advanced age, intoxication with illicit substances, some medications, other neurologic abnormalities, and cerebral ischemia. Some other important factors that can affect the readings include the timing after the injury and the technical quality of the recording. Although quantitative and conventional EEG may be useful as a supportive tool in the assessment of persons with concussion, the available evidence leaves uncertainty about whether applying this assessment method to the diagnosis of concussion represents a wise use of resources.[29]

VIRTUAL REALITY

Virtual reality testing creates a computer-simulated environment that is meant to mimic real-life situations and could potentially be used on the sidelines to assess the potential effects of concussion. The athlete should feel like they are inside the environment (presence) and that they have a sense of forward motion.[30] Some advantages that virtual reality testing have over other forms of testing are that it allows the athlete to experience the situation in a three-dimensional environment and it is a more accurate simulation of the real-life situations. A device (hardware) is placed over the athlete's eyes and creates a moving room experience (software). A sensor located on the athlete's head allows real-time tracking of position, orientation in yaw, pitch, and roll directions. Virtual reality testing has the capability to measure spatial memory, balance, reaction time, attention, and recall memory. A recent study at Pennsylvania State University found that virtual reality testing validly measures postural stability and that the nature of the test is capable of detecting balance deficits associated with postconcussive injury.[31] However, there is still the need for further testing to determine if virtual reality testing is a valid and reproducible modality to use for sideline assessment of concussion. Also, in comparison with other tools used to assess the effects of concussion, virtual reality testing has a much higher cost.

HEAD IMPACT SENSORS

Head impact sensors are devices inserted into mouth guards, helmets, or patches that enable the measurement of impact force and acceleration during sporting events. There is thought that there may be a certain force threshold or accumulation of forces that can lead to injury (concussion).[32] By monitoring these forces applied to the head during competition, these devices can alert the sideline staff that a potential significant event has occurred. The sensors also have the ability to follow the number, forces, and location of head impacts over a specific amount of time allowing the cataloging of their cumulative hits. The head impact telemetry system was developed at Virginia Tech and Dartmouth. It consists of electrodes that are inserted into the padding of a football helmet.[32] Another company, X2 Biosystems, Inc (Seattle, WA), has developed a sensor that is worn as a patch behind the mastoid. The patch can measure impact and also acceleration in multiple planes.[32] There is also the additional benefit of being applicable in multiple sports including those that do not require a helmet. The National Football League has recently adopted this technology for its teams. The X2 system allows real-time feedback to sideline personnel via a cloud-based server that is relayed to mobile devices. The evidence behind the use of these devices to monitor and diagnose concussion is lacking at this point and is a potential area for further research.[32]

NEUROPSYCHIATRIC TESTING

Neuropsychiatric testing has been a mainstay of concussion assessment for many years in a paper/pencil form and a computerized form. There are many different versions of computerized neuropsychiatric tests including the following:

- XLNTbrain Sport (XLNTbrain, National Harbor, MD)
- Computerized cognitive assessment tool (Axon Sports, Wausau, WI)
- Concussion resolution index (HeadMinder, Inc, New York, NY)
- Automated neuropsychological assessment metrics system (Washington, DC)
- Concussion vital signs (CNS Vital Signs, Morrisville, NC)

The most commonly used computerized neuropsychiatric test is the immediate postconcussion assessment and cognitive testing (ImPACT) developed at the University of Pittsburgh Medical Center. Now available as an application on smartphones and tablets, it has the potential for use on the sidelines. The test takes about 25 minutes (severely limiting sideline utility) to complete and measures multiple areas of cognitive functioning including

- Attention span
- Working memory
- Sustained and selective attention time
- Response variability
- Nonverbal problem solving
- Reaction time

The test itself consists of the following six modules:

- Word discrimination
- Design memory
- Xs and Os
- Symbol matching
- Color matching
- Three-letter memory

Composite scores are recorded in four categories: (1) memory composite verbal, (2) memory composite visual, (3) visual motor speed composite, and (4) reaction time composite. The raw scores from each of these categories are tabulated and a percentile score is given. Ideally, the scores are compared with a recent asymptomatic baseline of the athlete. If a baseline is not accurate then it is possible to compare the score with the more than 5 million baseline tests that have been done in the past.[33] There have been many studies done assessing the use of ImPACT in the diagnosis and management of athletes with concussion. Some studies have shown that it is sufficiently sensitive and specific to be used in the evaluation of the concussed athlete.[34] However, it has been criticized for being limited in its scope compared with other neuropsychiatric tests.[35] In addition, there is the potential for athletes to "sandbag" or intentionally score poorly on their baseline making the interpretation of scores after a potential event more difficult. The general consensus is that ImPACT is one of many tools that can be used to diagnose and treat concussion, but it should never be used alone in diagnosis and return-to-play decisions.

DISCUSSION/SUMMARY

The diagnosis of concussion can often be difficult to make. The sideline assessment of concussion is further complicated by environmental conditions and the time constraints that are often present. There are many tools and tests available to assist in the sideline evaluation of concussion. These tools and tests provide the ability to assess the athlete in four different areas: (1) associated symptoms, (2) cognitive ability, (3) balance, and (4) visual tracking.

Ideally these tests and tools should be inexpensive, simple to administer, reliable, reproducible, and time sensitive. It is ideal if the test is used by health professionals and nonhealth professionals (coaches and parents). It is recognized that the SCAT3, which incorporates the SAC, modified BESS, Maddocks questions, and coordination testing, is probably the most reliable and thorough sideline tool at this time. The King-Devick test is an easily applied sideline test that can be used by parents and coaches when athletic trainers or team physicians are not available. There are other tools, such as head impact sensors, EEG, and computerized neuropsychiatric testing, although each of these options either show conflicting support or have not been validated. Concussion research is constantly changing and adapting making it important to continually adapt to new evidence.

REFERENCES

1. McCrory P, Meeuwisse WH, Aubry M, et al. Consensus statement on concussion in sport: the 4th International Conference on Concussion in Sport, Zurich, November 2012. J Athl Train 2013;48(4):554–75.
2. Daneshvar DH, Nowinski CJ, McKee AC, et al. The epidemiology of sports-related concussion. Clin Sports Med 2011;30(1):1–17, vii.
3. Harmon KG, Drezner JA, Gammons M. American Medical Society for Sports Medicine position statement: concussion in sport. Br J Sports Med 2013;47: 15–26.
4. Guskiewicz KM, McCrea M, Marshall SW, et al. Cumulative effects associated with recurrent concussion in collegiate football players: the NCAA concussion study. JAMA 2003;290:2549–55.
5. Kristman VL, Tator CH, Kreiger N, et al. Does the apolipoprotein epsilon 4 allele predispose varsity athletes to concussion? A prospective cohort study. Clin J Sport Med 2008;18(4):322–8.
6. Covassin T, Swanik CB, Sachs ML. Sex differences and the incidence of concussions among collegiate athletes. J Athl Train 2003;38:238–44.
7. Gessel LM, Fields SK, Collins CL, et al. Concussions among United States high school and collegiate athletes. J Athl Train 2007;42:495–503.
8. McCrea M, Hammeke T, Olsen G, et al. Unreported concussion in high school football players: implications for prevention. Clin J Sport Med 2004;14:13–7.
9. Torres DM, Galetta KM, Phillips HW. Sports-related concussion: anonymous survey of a collegiate cohort. Neurol Clin Pract 2013;3(4):279–87.
10. Guskiewicz KM, Marshall SW, Bailes J, et al. Recurrent concussion and risk of depression in retired professional football players. Med Sci Sports Exerc 2007; 39:903–9.
11. Alla S, Sullivan SJ, Hale L, et al. Self-report scales/checklists for the measurement of concussion symptoms: a systematic review. Br J Sports Med 2009;43(Suppl 1):i3–12.
12. Lovell MR, Iverson GL, Collins MW, et al. Measurement of symptoms following sports-related concussion: reliability and normative data for the post-concussion scale. Appl Neuropsychol 2006;13(3):166–74.
13. Maroon JC, Lovell MR, Norwig J, et al. Cerebral concussion in athletes: evaluation and neuropsychological testing. Neurosurgery 2000;47(3):659–69.

14. Maddocks DL, Dicker GD, Saling MM. The assessment of orientation following concussion in athletes. Clin J Sport Med 1995;5(1):32–5.
15. McCrea M. Standardized mental status testing on the sideline after sport-related concussion. J Athl Train 2001;36(3):274–9.
16. McCrea M, Kelly JP, Kluge J, et al. Standardized assessment of concussion in football players. Neurology 1997;48(3):586–8.
17. Ragan BG, Herrmann SD, Kang M, et al. Psychometric evaluation of the standardized assessment of concussion: evaluation of baseline validity using item analysis. Athletic Train Sports Health Care 2009;1(4):180–7.
18. Guskiewicz KM. Postural stability assessment following concussion: one piece of the puzzle. Clin J Sport Med 2001;11(3):182–9.
19. Burk JM, Munkasy BA, Joyner AB, et al. Balance error scoring system performance changes after a competitive athletic season. Clin J Sport Med 2013; 23(4):312–7.
20. Bell DR, Guskiewicz KM, Clark MA, et al. Systematic review of the balance error scoring system. Sports Health 2011;3(3):287–95.
21. Guskiewicz KM, Register-Mihalik J, McCrory P, et al. Evidence-based approach to revising the SCAT2: introducing the SCAT3. Br J Sports Med 2013;47(5): 289–93.
22. Jinguji TM, Bompadre V, Harmon KG, et al. Sport concussion assessment tool-2: baseline values for high school athletes. Br J Sports Med 2012;46:365–70.
23. Yeh JR, Hsu LC, Lin C, et al. Nonlinear analysis of sensory organization test for subjects with unilateral vestibular dysfunction. PLoS One 2014;9(3):e91230.
24. Broglio SP, Puetz TW. The effect of sport concussion on neurocognitive function, self-report symptoms and postural control: a meta-analysis. Sports Med 2008; 38(1):53–67.
25. Galetta KM, Morganroth J, Moehringer N, et al. Adding vision to concussion testing: a prospective study of sideline testing in youth and collegiate athletes. J Neuroophthalmol 2015;35(3):235–41.
26. Galetta KM, Brandes LE, Maki K, et al. The King-Devick test and sports-related concussion: study of a rapid visual screening tool in a collegiate cohort. J Neurol Sci 2011;309(1–2):34–9.
27. Eckner JT, Whitacre RD, Kirsch NL, et al. Evaluating a clinical measure of reaction time: an observational study. Percept Mot Skills 2009;108(3):717–20.
28. Eckner JT, Kutcher JS, Richardson JK. Effect of concussion on clinically measured reaction time in 9 NCAA Division I collegiate athletes: a preliminary study. PM R 2011;3(3):212–8.
29. Pacifico A, Amyot F, Arciniegas D, et al. A review of the effectiveness of neuroimaging modalities for the detection of traumatic brain injury. J Neurotrauma 2015;32(22):1693–721.
30. Slobounov SM, Slobounov ES, Newell KM. Application of virtual reality graphics in assessment of concussion. Cyberpsychol Behav 2006;9:188–91.
31. Teel EF, Slobounov SM. Validation of a virtual reality balance module for use in clinical concussion assessment and management. Clin J Sport Med 2015; 25(2):144–8.
32. Okonkwo DO, Tempel ZJ, Maroon J, et al. Sideline assessment tools for the evaluation of concussion in athletes: a review. Neurosurgery 2014;75(4): 582–95.
33. Iverson GL, Lovell MR, Collins MW. Interpreting change on ImPACT following sport concussion. Clin Neuropsychol 2003;17(4):460–7.

34. Schatz P, Pardini JE, Lovell MR, et al. Sensitivity and specificity of the ImPACT test battery for concussion in athletes. Arch Clin Neuropsychol 2006;21(1):91–9.
35. Maerlender A, Flashman L, Kessler A, et al. Examination of the construct validity of ImPACT computerized test, traditional, and experimental neuropsychological measures. Clin Neuropsychol 2010;24(8):1309–25.

Neuroimaging of Concussion

Justin M. Honce, MD*, Eric Nyberg, MD, Isaac Jones, MD, Lidia Nagae, MD

KEYWORDS

- Concussion • mTBI • Magnetic resonance imaging • Diffusion tensor imaging
- Functional MRI • Spectroscopy

KEY POINTS

- There is a strong need to develop objective measures to ensure accurate and timely diagnosis of concussion and mild traumatic brain injury (mTBI) and to guide subsequent management decisions. Neuroimaging is likely to play an important role in this process.
- Despite the superior soft tissue contrast available by MRI, computed tomography (CT) remains the first-line imaging modality of choice in the acute setting due to its speed, ubiquitous availability, lower cost, and infrequent contraindications precluding the need for screening procedures.
- Although microstructural sequelae of concussion/mTBI are mostly below the threshold for standard CT and conventional MRI techniques, advanced MRI techniques (diffusion tensor imaging, functional MRI, perfusion, spectroscopy) and PET provide insight into these injuries.

INTRODUCTION

The phenomenon of concussion has received increasing attention in recent years primarily due to increased awareness of sports-related concussion (SRC) in adolescent and professional athletes, and in military personnel. The incidence of SRC is estimated at 1.6 to 3.8 million annually,[1] and during the wars in Iraq and Afghanistan, up to 25,000 mild traumatic brain injuries (mTBIs) were reported each year in the US Armed forces.[2] It is estimated that direct medical costs and indirect costs, such as lost productivity related to concussion and mTBI, total $12 billion per year in the United States alone.[3] This increased attention and the substantial societal costs have led to the recent publication of new or updated practice guidelines and position statements from multiple medical and professional societies addressing the prevention,

None of the authors have any commercial or financial conflict of interest and no funding was received for this or related work.
Department of Radiology, University of Colorado School of Medicine, 12700 East 19th Avenue, Mailstop C278, Aurora, CO 80045, USA
* Corresponding author.
E-mail address: justin.honce@ucdenver.edu

diagnosis, and management of concussion.[4–8] The variations in these guidelines make clear that there is still a need to develop objective measures to ensure accurate and timely diagnosis of concussion and to guide subsequent management decisions. Neuroimaging is likely to play an important role in this process.

Concussion and mTBI labels are often used interchangeably; however, they should be considered distinct entities, at least for now.[6,9,10] According to the 4th International Conference on Concussion in Sport, concussion is defined as the syndrome resulting from low-velocity injuries to the head that result in clinical symptoms but do not demonstrate visible structural abnormalities on conventional neuroimaging studies.[6] Symptoms, which include headaches, dizziness, blurry vision, and difficulty concentrating typically, demonstrate rapid onset and are relatively short lived. mTBI is characterized by greater clinical symptoms and demonstrates some evidence of structural injury on conventional neuroimaging studies, but without the degree and duration of symptoms that would qualify as moderate TBI. Thus, concussion and mTBI occupy adjacent positions on the spectrum of TBI, with similar and overlapping clinical symptoms and distinguished by the presence or absence of findings on conventional neuroimaging. How long this differentiation will last is uncertain as more sensitive MRI techniques and higher magnet field strengths become available for clinical use, allowing for the detection of subtle injuries not visible with older techniques.[11,12] As such, in this review we discuss the literature regarding both concussion and mTBI.

When athletes or military personnel experience concussive symptoms, there are 2 major questions that need to be answered acutely. The question of most immediate importance is whether there is an associated structural abnormality, such as intracranial hemorrhage or fracture, which may need immediate intervention. These are typically detected by computed tomography (CT). The second major question to be addressed is what is the appropriate time to return to play or return to active duty. This decision is not trivial given that were a new head injury to occur before the symptoms of the previous injury have resolved, there is increased risk of severe brain injury and potentially death, even in the setting of a relatively mild trauma. This is known as "second impact syndrome."[13] Currently, the decision to return to the field is guided by symptoms and various sideline assessment tools,[14] but there is potential for neuroimaging techniques to help guide these decisions, both acutely and in the long term.

In this review, we focus on the role for neuroimaging in the concussed patient and describe the recommended practices related to imaging in concussion. This discussion first focuses on the exclusion of severe injuries and is followed by a discussion of the potential utility of various advanced imaging techniques in research and clinical practice.

DECIDING WHEN/IF TO IMAGE THE CONCUSSED PATIENT

Consensus recommendations from the 4th International Conference on Concussion in Sport, the American Medical Society for Sports Medicine, the American Academy of Neurology Concussion Guidelines, and the American College of Emergency Medicine/Centers for Disease Control and Prevention joint practice guidelines recommend that head CT be performed for individuals with more than 30 seconds of loss of consciousness, prolonged altered mental status, severe headache, focal neurologic deficits, or seizure.[4–6,15] There is, however, substantial overlap in the clinical symptoms of patients both with and without radiologically evident acute traumatic injuries on CT, and patients may be found to have acute intracranial findings on head CT in the setting of an unimpressive examination.[16] An additional consideration is the radiation dose from imaging. Most relevant is the stochastic effect, which is the likelihood of radiation exposure inducing cancer. Routine CT of the brain has an effective dose of 2 mSv and 1 CT brain scan is estimated to increase the lifetime risk of cancer by 0.016% in men and 0.026% in women.[17] As such, is it ultimately up to the clinical judgment of the caregiver whether or not to proceed to imaging, weighing the benefits of imaging against the costs, including financial costs and radiation exposure.

STRUCTURAL IMAGING: EXCLUDING ACUTE TRAUMATIC BRAIN INJURIES

In the past, conventional plain film radiography of the skull had a role in the diagnosis of skull fractures after head injury; however, this has been essentially supplanted by CT. Despite the superior soft tissue contrast available by MRI, CT remains the first-line imaging modality of choice due to its speed, ubiquitous availability, lower cost, and infrequent contraindications precluding the need for screening procedures.[18]

Computed Tomography

CT scanning uses a rotating x-ray tube and rotating x-ray detectors that measure x-ray attenuation and process detector data into gray-scale images. CT is highly sensitive for the detection of calvarial and facial fractures, as well as hemorrhage in the epidural, subdural, subarachnoid, intraventricular, and parenchymal spaces. It is also moderately sensitive to cerebral contusions that may or may not require neurosurgical intervention.[19,20] The precise incidence of traumatic intracranial injuries in the setting of SRC is not available, but there are some data on patients with mTBI of all causes. The literature shows variable rates of injury detected on CT, between 16% and 21% in one study of 912 patients with mTBI,[16] but as low as 3% and as high as 34% in other studies.[21,22] Acute injuries necessitating neurosurgical intervention, however, are low across studies, approximately 1% or less.[21–24] The sensitivity for detecting both skull fractures and subtle intraparenchymal and extra-axial hemorrhages can be improved by thin collimation acquisition using both 2-dimensional (2D) multiplanar and 3D reconstructions[25,26] **(Fig. 1)**.

Magnetic Resonance Imaging

MRI also has a role in imaging selected patients with suspected head trauma in the acute setting. As opposed to CT, MRI does not depend on ionizing radiation, but instead uses a strong magnetic field and radiofrequency pulses to excite spinning protons in tissues to create imaging with numerous different tissue contrasts. Given its higher cost and other limitations, MRI is typically reserved for patients in whom the initial CT was deemed negative but whose symptoms are not improving[27] or to further evaluate patients in whom the initial CT demonstrated brain injury.

MRI outperforms CT for the detection of parenchymal injuries, including diffuse axonal shear injury (DAI) and small parenchymal contusions **(Fig. 2)**. MRI is more sensitive than CT in the detection of subdural and epidural hematomas,[28–32] whereas CT is more sensitive to subarachnoid hemorrhage.[19,20] Fluid attenuated inversion recovery (FLAIR) imaging is particularly sensitive to parenchymal edema, allowing identification of small contusions that can be missed on CT. There is also excellent conspicuity of extra-axial hematomas on FLAIR MRI, allowing for the detection of thin hematomas, which can be inconspicuous on CT **(Fig. 3)**.[33] T2 star (T2*)-weighted gradient-echo imaging (GRE) exploits the distortions in magnetic fields created by paramagnetic material, which makes it exquisitely sensitive to blood products in certain stages of degradation. GRE is therefore very sensitive to the microhemorrhages associated with DAI. In patients with neurologic changes in the setting of rapid deceleration injury, for example, MRI should be performed, as DAI is frequently missed

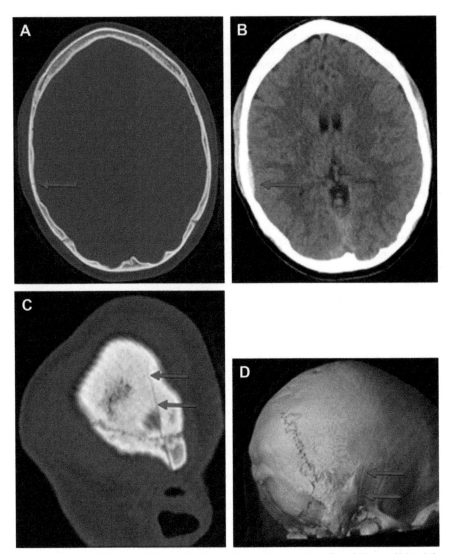

Fig. 1. A 25-year-old man with headache and vomiting 1 day after falling off his bike. Patient was originally evaluated by his primary care provider and diagnosed with concussion. (*A*) Axial CT image bone window) demonstrating a nondisplaced fracture through the right temporal bone (*red arrow*). (*B*) Axial CT image (brain and blood window) demonstrating a shallow underlying epidural hematoma (*red arrow*). (*C*) Sagittal multiplanar reformat and (*D*) 3D reconstruction nicely display the length of the fracture (*red arrows*).

on CT (**Fig. 4**).[32,34–37] Susceptibility-weighted imaging (SWI), a newer iteration using the susceptibility principle, further increases sensitivity for susceptibility-related signal, resulting in greater susceptibility signal blooming and increased lesion conspicuity.[34,38] Although MRI is more sensitive for small lesions, severe injuries necessitating neurosurgical intervention are typically easily detected by either CT or MRI.[19,20,28]

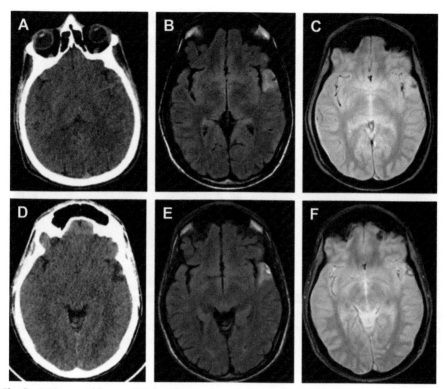

Fig. 2. A 29-year-old man with headache after a motor vehicle collision. (*A*) Axial CT image demonstrates subtle hemorrhage along the left temporal lobe (*red arrow*). (*B*) Axial FLAIR, and (*C*) axial T2* images demonstrating a left temporal lobe contusion with mild associated hemorrhage. (*D*) Axial CT, (*E*) FLAIR, and (*F*) T2* images 4 days later show maturation of the contusion, now conspicuous on CT as well as MR (*red arrow* in D).

The clinical utility of MRI for the detection of small areas of brain injury not visible on CT has recently been investigated. Yuh and colleagues,[39,40] in a multicenter prospective study of 135 consecutive patients with mTBI in the emergency department evaluated for acute head injury demonstrated that small parenchymal contusions or 4 or more sites of hemorrhagic shearing detected by MRI but not visible on CT were independent predictors of poorer 3-month outcome as measured by the Extended Glasgow Outcome Scale at 3 months after injury.

ADVANCED AND EXPERIMENTAL IMAGING TECHNIQUES FOR THE EVALUATION OF CONCUSSION

Concussion is generally believed to be a functional, rather than structural, brain injury, which develops when trauma to the head places the brain under translational and/or rotational acceleration-deceleration forces.[6,41–44] These forces result in injuries to cell membranes and ionic pumps, causing pathologic ionic cascades and loss of neurochemical homeostasis,[45] with resulting clinical symptoms. Although microstructural sequelae of most of these traumas are below the threshold for standard CT and conventional MRI techniques, more advanced MR techniques are being developed to assess the full extent of injury. These techniques include ultra-high field structural

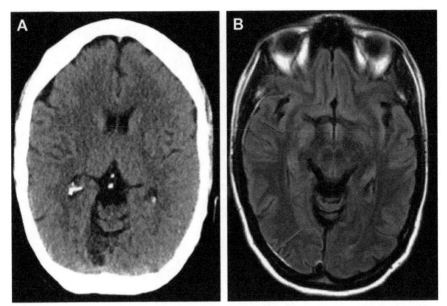

Fig. 3. A 45-year-old man with a headache after a fall. The initial CT brain study (*A*) was normal. (*B*) Given the lack of improvement in symptoms, an MRI was obtained 1 week later demonstrating thin extra-axial hyperintensity on FLAIR (*arrows*), consistent with a small subdural hematoma.

imaging, diffusion tensor imaging (DTI), functional MRI (fMRI), perfusion imaging, PET scanning, and magnetic resonance spectroscopy (MRS).

Ultra-High Field Structural Imaging

MRI is typically performed with 1.5 T (1.5 T) or 3.0 T magnetic field strengths and conventional MRI sequences including GRE, SWI, and FLAIR show improved sensitivity at

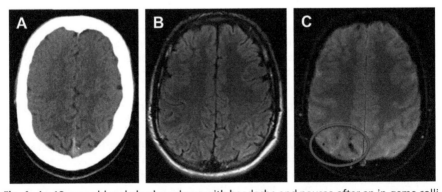

Fig. 4. An 18-year-old male hockey player with headache and nausea after an in-game collision. (*A*) Axial CT image obtained at presentation is normal. (*B*) Follow-up FLAIR imaging from the same examination is also normal. (*C*) However, MRI T2* image shows multiple small parenchymal hemorrhages within the right parietal subcortical white matter consistent with shear injury and diffuse axonal injury (*red circled outline*).

3.0 T versus 1.5 T. Ultra-high field MRI at field strengths of 7 T and beyond is being investigated for use in detection of microstructural traumatic injuries, although this is not in widespread clinical use. One study assessing the performance of SWI at 7 T and 3 T in patients with mTBI found that at 7 T up to 41% more microhemorrhagic shearing injuries were identified than at 3 T, and the shearing injuries visible at 3 T were shown to be significantly larger at 7 T.[46] The 7-T MRI may also improve tissue specificity, with one preliminary study showing that in some cases of concussion, suspected shearing injuries visible at 3 T were found to be developmental venous anomalies at 7 T.[11] The greatly increased detection of microstructural injury in the setting of mTBI may eventually lead to a redefinition of concussion as a microstructural traumatic derangement, rather than a purely "functional" phenomenon, although this has yet to be demonstrated.

Diffusion Tensor Imaging

Diffusion-weighted imaging (DWI) is a specialized imaging sequence that images the Brownian motion of water molecules as they diffuse through the extracellular space, irrespective of the direction of diffusion. DTI builds on DWI by characterizing the directionality of the diffusion of water in 3D space by measuring the diffusion in at least 6 different directions, but potentially up to hundreds.[47] Given that the diffusion of water is highly influenced by tissue microstructure, DTI is especially useful for measuring the microstructural integrity of highly ordered tissues, such as the white matter, via fractional anisotropy (FA).[48,49] FA is represented as a value between 0 and 1, in which 0 indicates a completely isotropic environment in which there is no restriction to diffusion in any direction, and 1, in which water is capable of diffusing in only 1 axis. White matter in the commissures, such as the corpus callosum, typically have FA values between 0.6 and 0.8, but FA in the rest of the white matter is typically lower[47,50] (**Fig. 5**). Besides FA, other DTI parameters can be evaluated, including mean diffusivity (MD), which is overall magnitude of the diffusivity; radial diffusivity (RD), which is the diffusivity perpendicular to a fiber bundle; and axial diffusivity (AD), which is the diffusivity along the fiber bundle. There has been some suggestion that RD may be more specific

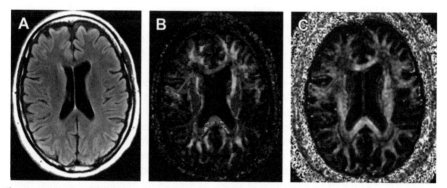

Fig. 5. A 56-year-old woman with a history of multiple minor head injuries and recent fall with persistent complaints of mental fogginess, sleep disturbance, and fatigue. (*A*) Axial FLAIR image is unremarkable other than mild diffuse volume loss. (*B*) Color DTI map demonstrates white matter tracts with color-coded orientation (red, transverse; blue, craniocaudad; green, anterior-posterior). (*C*) Axial FA image demonstrates the FA as gray-scale values (dark low FA, white high FA). Color DTI (*B*) and FA (*C*) images demonstrate decreased tensor density and FA in the right side of the genu of the corpus callosum (*red arrows*), presumably posttraumatic.

to myelin damage, and AD more specific to axonal damage,[51–53] but this is probably a convenient generalization made in the early stage of a rapidly developing field.

DTI may be a valuable tool for assessment of patients with concussion and mTBI. Numerous studies have described changes in various DTI metrics following concussion and TBI, typically in patients in the subacute or later stages from the initial injury and with persistent symptoms.[49,54–72] The results of these studies vary, with many showing reduced FA or increased MD, indicative of microstructural damage in concussion and patients with mTBI compared with controls; however, other studies show the opposite findings, with elevated FA or decreased MD,[55,62,67,70] whereas still others show mixed or no differences.[56,63,66] Microstructural abnormalities in these studies are found widely throughout the brain, including the anterior and posterior corpus callosum, internal capsules, frontal and parietal corona radiata, and the uncinate fasciculus. Some studies also showed that alterations in diffusivity correlate with the severity of postconcussive symptoms.[65,69] These studies demonstrate group differences in DTI parameters, making their applicability in the individual patient of little use. There are ongoing efforts to assess the potential of DTI for prognostic purposes in individual patients. Yuh and colleagues,[73] in a recent study of 76 patients with mTBI, demonstrated reduced FA compared with control subjects and found that reduced FA was a significant predictor of both 3-month and 6-month outcomes measured by the Glasgow Outcome Scale. More work is needed before a consensus can be reached regarding the best way to use DTI for diagnosis and prognosis in individual patients.

Functional MRI

fMRI relies on the coupling of increased neuronal activity and compensatory changes in vascular perfusion to create maps of cerebral activity. When neurons activate, there is increased extraction of oxygen from local tissues, which triggers an overcompensating vasodilatory response that results in elevated levels of oxyhemoglobin and relatively decreased level of deoxyhemoglobin. This relative decrease in the amount of deoxyhemoglobin is measured through blood oxygen level–dependent (BOLD) imaging. BOLD fMRI can be performed either with task-based paradigms, or in the resting state.[74] During task-based BOLD fMRI, patients are imaged during alternating periods of task performance or stimulus presentation, and rest. Therefore, the differences in BOLD signal between the active and passive phases appear as regional activations associated with the task or stimulus. For resting state BOLD fMRI, subjects are imaged entirely at rest and the temporal relationships of spontaneous low-frequency variations in BOLD signal are used to assess the functional connectivity of various brain regions.[75]

Numerous studies have investigated patients with concussion and patients with mTBI with task-based fMRI. Most studies have used tasks that focus on working and declarative memory, attention, and other aspects of executive functioning.[56,76–84] Studies comparing symptomatic, concussed adult patients and healthy controls commonly demonstrate little or no differences in performance of functional tasks. On fMRI, adults with concussion demonstrate either abnormal hypo-activation or hyper-activation in regions related to executive functioning, such as the dorsolateral prefrontal cortex (DLPFC) and parietal lobes, as well as increased activation in more widely distributed brain regions, suggesting recruitment of these areas.[76–78,82,83] These functional abnormalities may persist for several months[78] but may eventually normalize.[77] This suggests that for a concussed individual to satisfactorily perform a given task, his or her brain may have to work harder, by engaging compensatory strategies that include increased alterations in activity in task-related regions and/or recruitment of more widespread brain regions than healthy controls. The picture in adolescents may be different. Keightley and colleagues[84] assessed 15 adolescents with concussion and 15 matched controls using BOLD fMRI and a standardized working memory task. In contradistinction to adults, concussed adolescents performed poorer on the task than controls, with reduced task related performance in the bilateral DLPFC, left premotor cortex, left superior parietal lobule, and other widely distributed regions. Interestingly, task performance was significantly correlated with signal changes in the DLPFC (greater DLPFC activation was associated with greater accuracy on the task). This finding, in the setting of reduced task performance and reduced activation in the DLPFC, suggests that unlike adults, concussed youths may be unable to adequately compensate to maintain cognitive performance. This may have implications in "return-to-play" decisions.

Resting state fMRI studies examining functional connectivity demonstrate decreased or increased connectivity between various brain regions after concussion.[85–89] Mayer and colleagues[87] have shown decreased functional connectivity within the default mode network (DMN) and hyperconnectivity between the DMN and lateral prefrontal cortex, and others have found both reduced connectivity in posterior regions of the DMN (posterior cingulate, parietal lobe) and increased connectivity in the anterior portions of the DMN (medial prefrontal cortex).[85] Abnormalities in numerous other functional networks, including those involved in cognitive and motor control and visual processing, also have been reported.[89] Obviously, findings are varied/mixed and limited conclusions can be drawn regarding the consistency and significance of these data, as most studies at this point have been limited by relatively small sample sizes and varying time points from injury.

Ultimately, both task-based and resting state fMRI have demonstrated group differences between patients with concussion/mTBI and controls. Although there is variation in the results, the major themes implicate dysfunction in executive functioning, particularly in the frontal lobes; youths are more likely to develop cognitive deficits than are adults; and that concussed subjects who perform comparably to controls may be able to compensate for the injury through recruitment of other brain regions supporting the given task.

Perfusion Imaging

Several studies using perfusion-imaging techniques have been performed in recent years to assess changes in regional blood flow, a surrogate for metabolism, in the brain in patients with mTBI and normal conventional brain imaging findings. These studies have demonstrated regional perfusion deficits that have correlated with posttraumatic cognitive and psychological impairment.[90] A variety of imaging techniques have been used in this regard, including perfusion CT, dynamic susceptibility contrast, and arterial spin-labeling (ASL) MR perfusion imaging, single-photon emission computed tomography (SPECT), and PET. No single modality has emerged as singularly more useful than the others in the evaluation of mTBI; the relative advantages and disadvantages of each modality are therefore discussed.

Perfusion computed tomography

Perfusion CT is performed by continuously scanning through the brain during the first pass of an intravenous contrast bolus. This yields time-density curves for each voxel from which cerebral blood volume (CBV), cerebral blood flow (CBF), mean transit time, and time to peak can be calculated.[91] Postprocessing software generates a complete set of parametric maps typically within a few minutes of completing a scan.[92]

In current clinical practice, perfusion CT is not routinely used in the evaluation of TBI. Perfusion CT is obtained in acute TBI, when there is suspected concurrent vascular injury and acute ischemic infarct. A few studies have investigated the utility of perfusion CT specifically for assessment of TBI, demonstrating a higher sensitivity for the diagnosis of cerebral contusions when compared with noncontrast CT at the time of hospital admission, with reported sensitivity of 87.5% versus 39.6%.[91] Additionally, these scans obtained in the acute phase were independently predictive of functional outcome at 3 to 6 months, with normal brain perfusion or hyperemia predicting favorable outcomes and oligemic patterns predictive of unfavorable outcomes.[91,93] The examination requires substantial radiation, however, and appropriate selection of patients who would benefit most from this examination is therefore critical.[90] Further studies will be required before the question of appropriateness is resolved.

Perfusion MRI

MRI is an appealing modality for assessment of perfusion abnormalities in mTBI/concussion given the lack of ionizing radiation, typically performed whether with dynamic susceptibility contrast (DSC) or arterial spin labeling (ASL). DSC is performed by measuring signal change during the first pass of an intravenous bolus of gadolinium-based contrast, and using the tissue concentration–time curves to generate maps of relative CBF and volume (rCBF and rCBV, respectively). ASL labels flowing blood with radiofrequency pulses creating an "endogenous contrast" that can be used to calculate CBF. ASL does not require an intravenous contrast agent, and is therefore completely noninvasive and repeatable. In addition, truly quantitative values of CBF can be obtained rather than relative values.[94] DSC, however, provides a higher signal-to-noise ratio and higher spatial resolution compared with ASL.

Only a few small studies have explored the utility of perfusion MRI for evaluation of mTBI with imaging primarily performed in the subacute to chronic phases of injury. Both DSC and ASL were able to detect reductions in relative CBF and CBVs within in various regions of the brain, which correlated with associated neurocognitive deficits.[95–97] Further research is required to determine the utility of these examinations in this setting.

Single-photon emission computed tomography

SPECT imaging involves injection of a radiopharmaceutical into the bloodstream, which then accumulates in regions of the body according to its biological properties. The most commonly used radiopharmaceuticals for SPECT imaging of the brain are technetium-99m-hexamethylpropyleneamine oxime (99mTc-HMPAO) and 99m Tc-ethyl cysteinate dimer. These radiotracers travel to regions of the brain proportional to perfusion and are taken up by brain cells.

Studies have shown SPECT perfusion imaging to be sensitive to mTBI, showing decreases in CBF to various areas of the brain and SPECT may be more sensitive compared with conventional CT or MRI in both the acute and chronic settings. Furthermore, SPECT lesion localizations have been shown to be concordant with neuropsychological tests.[98] SPECT has a strong negative predictive value, with TBI-associated symptoms resolving within 3 months in 89% to 97% of patients with negative SPECT examination within the first month following injury and 100% negative predictive value when performed at 1 year after injury.[99,100] Positive predictive value of SPECT increases over time with 59% of those with an abnormal SPECT in the first month after injury remaining symptomatic at 3-month follow-up, compared with 83% when imaged at 1 year after injury.[99,100] Although these results are promising, current limitations in the evidence to support the routine clinical use of SPECT perfusion imaging in the evaluation of mTBI include very few randomized controlled trials and various levels of analytical rigor used to identify TBI-associated changes with SPECT imaging.[90]

Positron Emission Tomography

PET is an imaging method that requires injection of a radiopharmaceutical, followed by scanning performed at a set interval. A wide variety of PET radiopharmaceuticals are available for brain studies, some of which include those used to image cerebral perfusion; glucose, protein, and oxygen metabolism; amyloid deposition; and neurotransmitter systems. PET has higher spatial resolution than SPECT and suffers from fewer artifacts, albeit at a higher cost.

Much of the research evaluating mTBI with PET has focused on identifying metabolic anomalies using 18F-Fluorodeoxyglucose (18-FDG). Global and focal alterations in glucose metabolism have been observed after mTBI.[101] A few small studies in the setting of chronic mTBI have shown correlation between findings on 18-FDG images and cognitive tests[102]; however, data should be considered preliminary and the literature is as yet inconclusive.

A recently developed compound, [18F]-fluoroethyl-methyl-amino-2-naphthylethylidene-malononitrile (FDDNP), has affinity for pathologic deposits of beta-amyloid and tau protein, both of which are found in various neurodegenerative diseases. This compound may potentially serve as a marker for chronic traumatic encephalopathy (CTE), which is believed to be a progressive tauopathy, found in individuals who have had repetitive concussive brain injuries.[103] Currently, there is no definitive clinical diagnosis of CTE, and as such it would benefit from a method of early diagnosis, particularly for the development of experimental therapeutic interventions. Preliminary investigations have demonstrated promise for this radiopharmaceutical while research is currently ongoing.[104] Another newer compound, [18F]-THK523, shows promise as a tau-specific marker.[105]

Magnetic Resonance Spectroscopy

Metabolites may be identified by their chemical shift resonance in MRI, expressed in parts per million (ppm), independent of the field strength used. In the brain, N-acetyl aspartate (NAA, at 2.01 ppm) is a marker of neuronal population and function; total choline (Cho, at 3.2 ppm), including primarily phosphoryl and glycerophosphoryl choline, reflects turnover of membranes; creatine (Cr, at 3.0 ppm), composed of phosphocreatine, is considered a reference value related to energetic metabolism; myo-inositol (ml, at 3.56 ppm) is related to glial proliferation; glutamate/glutamine complex (Glx, at 2.12–2.35 and 3.74–3.75 ppm) is the major excitatory neurotransmitter in the brain; and lactate (Lac, at 1.33 ppm) is related to anaerobic glycolysis. It is important to note that the levels of metabolites vary with the anatomic location evaluated and with aging.

As a noninvasive method capable of revealing the metabolic profile in the brain, MRS may be a suitable method for both initial diagnosis and longitudinal follow-up in SRC; however, this utility currently remains essentially restricted to research. Various combinations of metabolites identified by single-voxel or multivoxel techniques may potentially reveal the neurometabolic imbalance of inflammatory and excitatory cascade metabolites related to the pathophysiology of trauma. In the acute setting of SRC (1–6 days), decreased NAA has been demonstrated in the frontal lobes, which was correlated with self-reported symptoms and/or neuropsychological testing results, with variable deficits in attention, verbal memory, visual memory, information-processing speed, and reaction time.[106,107] Decreased Cr and ml levels in the DLPFC and decreased Glx in the primary motor (M1) region have been found in nondiagnosed asymptomatic collision high school football athletes over the season, reflecting ongoing metabolic disturbance despite lack of clinically reportable symptoms.[108]

Decreased NAA/Cr and NAA/Cho ratios are believed to reflect impaired energetic metabolism, occurring during the post concussive vulnerable period of the brain. This window of vulnerability to a second minor trauma leading to second-impact syndrome has been demonstrated by MRS.[109,110] Three days after concussion, decreased NAA/Cr and NAA/Cho ratios in bilateral frontal white matter were shown to return to normal after 30 days in athletes who suspended practice, as opposed to after 45 days in athletes who had a second concussion within 15 days of the first one. Reported resolution of symptoms was between 3 and 15 days for the patients with a single concussion and at 30 days for the patients with repeat concussion, earlier than the resolution of MRS changes. Variability in the levels of Cr, originally thought to be constant in the brain, has also been demonstrated on longitudinal SRC studies, perhaps reflecting decreased energy metabolism levels seen in more severe cases.[111] Demonstration of increased mI/Cr and Glx/Cr levels in the M1 region in concussed football athletes after 6 months of injury, not present in the acute phase, suggests metabolic derangement as a dynamic process that may evolve over time.[112]

SUMMARY

Concussion and mTBI are serious issues with substantial socioeconomic and personal costs for adolescent and professional athletes and military personnel. The main role for neuroimaging in the clinical setting is the exclusion of serious intracranial injuries, some of which may warrant neurosurgical intervention. CT is the first-line modality in the workup of patients with head injury and can typically rule out severe traumatic injury necessitating neurosurgical intervention. However, MRI is becoming increasingly available and is more sensitive than CT for subtle hemorrhagic and nonhemorrhagic cerebral injuries. With increased utilization of higher field strength MRI and more sensitive and specialized sequences, microstructural and functional abnormalities not detectable with older technologies are increasingly detected. These new imaging techniques are improving our understanding of concussion and the associated underlying microstructural, functional, metabolic, and perfusion derangements.

A multitude of imaging modalities and techniques are currently under exploration to address the diverse clinical questions and scenarios discussed in this article; however, the "Holy Grail" of imaging in any setting is to be able to address virtually all of the clinical questions associated with that setting, in this case trauma. Although each imaging modality has its specific strengths, only MRI has the breadth to address most of the issues discussed in this article. MRI technology is highly sensitive to blood products in the acute, subacute, and chronic settings, including the detection of acute microhemorrhages not detected elsewhere; is exquisitely sensitive to both intracellular and extracellular edema; has the unique ability to detect derangement in the microstructure of white matter tracts; can perform perfusion analysis without the need for intravenous contrast; and can query chemical and metabolite abnormalities with MRS. The authors look forward to a time when the full known potential of MRI can be routinely (and affordably) used in the service of most or all patients suffering from mTBI or moderate TBI in the acute setting, thus enabling a more informed triage algorithm and clinical interventions. Although these specialized techniques are currently predominantly reserved for research,[90] they may come to play a significant role in improving diagnosis, prognosis, and improvement in such key management decisions as when it is safe to return to play or active duty.

REFERENCES

1. Langlois JA, Rutland-Brown W, Wald MM. The epidemiology and impact of traumatic brain injury: a brief overview. J Head Trauma Rehabil 2006;21:375–8.
2. Defense.gov. Special report: traumatic brain injury. Available at: http://www.defense.gov/home/features/2012/0312_tbi/. Accessed August, 2015.
3. CDC. CDC | TBI Data and Statistics | Traumatic Brain Injury | Injury Center. Available at: http://www.cdc.gov/traumaticbraininjury/data/index.html. Accessed August, 2015.
4. Harmon KG, Drezner JA, Gammons M, et al. American Medical Society for Sports Medicine position statement: concussion in sport. Br J Sports Med 2013;47:15–26.
5. Giza CC, Kutcher JS, Ashwal S, et al. Summary of evidence-based guideline update: evaluation and management of concussion in sports Report of the Guideline Development Subcommittee of the American Academy of Neurology. Neurology 2013;80:2250–7.
6. McCrory P, Meeuwisse WH, Aubry M, et al. Consensus statement on concussion in sport: the 4th International Conference on Concussion in Sport held in Zurich, November 2012. Br J Sports Med 2013;47:250–8.
7. NFL Head, Neck and Spine Committee's Protocols Regarding Diagnosis and Management of Concussion. NFL Players Association 2013. Available at: http://images.nflplayers.com/mediaResources/lyris/pdfs/NFL_Diagnosis_Mgmt_Concussion.pdf. Accessed August, 2015.
8. Veterans Affairs / Department of Defense Clinical Practice Guidelines: Management of Concussion / Mild Traumatic Injury. Available at: http://www.healthquality.va.gov/guidelines/Rehab/mtbi/. Accessed August, 2015.
9. Dimou S, Lagopoulos J. Toward objective markers of concussion in sport: a review of white matter and neurometabolic changes in the brain after sports-related concussion. J Neurotrauma 2013;31:413–24.
10. McCrory P, Meeuwisse WH, Echemendia RJ, et al. What is the lowest threshold to make a diagnosis of concussion? Br J Sports Med 2013;47:268–71.
11. Russman A, Figler R, Oh S-H, et al. 7 tesla brain MRI characteristics among concussion patients (P7.162). Neurology 2015;84:P7–162.
12. Bazarian JJ, Blyth B, Cimpello L. Bench to bedside: evidence for brain injury after concussion—looking beyond the computed tomography scan. Acad Emerg Med 2006;13:199–214.
13. Dessy AM, Rasouli J, Choudhri TF. Second impact syndrome: a rare, devastating consequence of repetitive head injuries. Neurosurg Q 2015;25:423–6.
14. Okonkwo DO, Tempel ZJ, Maroon J. Sideline assessment tools for the evaluation of concussion in athletes: a review. Neurosurgery 2014;75:S82–95.
15. Jagoda AS, Bazarian JJ, Bruns JJ Jr, et al. Clinical policy: neuroimaging and decisionmaking in adult mild traumatic brain injury in the acute setting. Ann Emerg Med 2008;52:714–48.
16. Iverson GL, Lovell MR, Smith S, et al. Prevalence of abnormal CT-scans following mild head injury. Brain Inj 2000;14:1057–61.
17. BEIR VII. Committee to Assess Health Risks From Exposure to Low Levels of Ionizing Radiation. Health Risks From Exposure to Low Levels of Ionizing Radiation. BEIR VII. Washington, DC: National Research Council; 2006.
18. Ginde AA, Foianini A, Renner DM, et al. Availability and quality of computed tomography and magnetic resonance imaging equipment in U.S. emergency departments. Acad Emerg Med 2008;15:780–3.

19. Gentry LR, Godersky JC, Thompson B, et al. Prospective comparative study of intermediate-field Mr and CT in the evaluation of closed head trauma. AJR Am J Neuroradiol 1988;9:91–100.

20. Orrison WW, Gentry LR, Stimac GK, et al. Blinded comparison of cranial CT and MR in closed head injury evaluation. AJR Am J Neuroradiol 1994;15:351–6.

21. Thiruppathy SP, Muthukumar N. Mild head injury: revisited. Acta Neurochir (Wien) 2004;146:1075–82 [discussion: 1082–3].

22. Nagy KK, Joseph KT, Krosner SM, et al. The utility of head computed tomography after minimal head injury. J Trauma 1999;46:268–70.

23. Borg J, Holm L, Cassidy JD, et al. Diagnostic procedures in mild traumatic brain injury: results of the WHO collaborating centre task force on mild traumatic brain injury. J Rehabil Med 2004;36:61–75.

24. af Geijerstam JL, Britton M. Mild head injury–mortality and complication rate: meta-analysis of findings in a systematic literature review. Acta Neurochir (Wien) 2003;145:843–50.

25. Zacharia TT, Nguyen DTD. Subtle pathology detection with multidetector row coronal and sagittal CT reformations in acute head trauma. Emerg Radiol 2009;17:97–102.

26. Orman G, Wagner MW, Seeburg D, et al. Pediatric skull fracture diagnosis: should 3D CT reconstructions be added as routine imaging? J Neurosurg Pediatr 2015;16(4):426–31.

27. Yuh EL, Hawryluk GWJ, Manley GT. Imaging concussion: a review. Neurosurgery 2014;75:S50–63.

28. Kelly AB, Zimmerman RD, Snow RB, et al. Head trauma: comparison of MR and CT–experience in 100 patients. AJR Am J Neuroradiol 1988;9:699–708.

29. Jenkins A, Hadley MDM, Teasdale G, et al. Brain lesions detected by magnetic resonance imaging in mild and severe head injuries. Lancet 1986;328:445–6.

30. Mittl RL, Grossman RI, Hiehle JF, et al. Prevalence of MR evidence of diffuse axonal injury in patients with mild head injury and normal head CT findings. AJR Am J Neuroradiol 1994;15:1583–9.

31. Lee H, Wintermark M, Gean AD, et al. Focal lesions in acute mild traumatic brain injury and neurocognitive outcome: CT versus 3T MRI. J Neurotrauma 2008;25:1049–56.

32. Beauchamp MH, Ditchfield M, Babl FE, et al. Detecting traumatic brain lesions in children: CT versus MRI versus susceptibility weighted imaging (SWI). J Neurotrauma 2011;28:915–27.

33. Morais DF, Spotti AR, Tognola WA, et al. Clinical application of magnetic resonance in acute traumatic brain injury. Arq Neuropsiquiatr 2008;66:53–8.

34. Tong KA, Ashwal S, Holshouser BA, et al. Hemorrhagic shearing lesions in children and adolescents with posttraumatic diffuse axonal injury: improved detection and initial results. Radiology 2003;227:332–9.

35. Ashwal S, Tong KA, Ghosh N, et al. Application of advanced neuroimaging modalities in pediatric traumatic brain injury. J Child Neurol 2014;29:1704–17.

36. Mittal S, Wu Z, Neelavalli J, et al. Susceptibility-weighted imaging: technical aspects and clinical applications, part 2. AJR Am J Neuroradiol 2009;30:232–52.

37. Kuzma BB, Goodman JM. Improved identification of axonal shear injuries with gradient echo MR technique. Surg Neurol 2000;53:400–2.

38. Ashwal S, Babikian T, Gardner-Nichols J, et al. Susceptibility-weighted imaging and proton magnetic resonance spectroscopy in assessment of outcome after pediatric traumatic brain injury. Arch Phys Med Rehabil 2006;87:50–8.

39. Yuh EL, Mukherjee P, Lingsma HF, et al. Magnetic resonance imaging improves 3-month outcome prediction in mild traumatic brain injury. Ann Neurol 2013;73: 224–35.

40. Yue JK, Vassar MJ, Lingsma HF, et al. Transforming research and clinical knowledge in traumatic brain injury pilot: multicenter implementation of the common data elements for traumatic brain injury. J Neurotrauma 2013;30:1831–44.

41. Holbourn AHS. Mechanics of head injuries. Lancet 1943;242:438–41.

42. Graham DI, Adams JH, Nicoll JAR, et al. The nature, distribution and causes of traumatic brain injury. Brain Pathol 1995;5:397–406.

43. Ommaya AK, Gennarelli TA. Cerebral concussion and traumatic unconsciousness. Brain 1974;97:633–54.

44. Denny-Brown D, Russell WR. Experimental cerebral concussion. Brain 1941;64: 93–164.

45. Katayama Y, Becker DP, Tamura T, et al. Massive increases in extracellular potassium and the indiscriminate release of glutamate following concussive brain injury. J Neurosurg 2009;112(Spec Suppl):889–900.

46. Moenninghoff C, Kraff O, Maderwald S, et al. Diffuse axonal injury at ultra-high field MRI. PLoS One 2015;10:e0122329.

47. Le Bihan D, Mangin JF, Poupon C, et al. Diffusion tensor imaging: concepts and applications. J Magn Reson Imaging 2001;13:534–46.

48. Basser PJ, Mattiello J, LeBihan D. MR diffusion tensor spectroscopy and imaging. Biophys J 1994;66:259–67.

49. Kraus MF, Susmaras T, Caughlin BP, et al. White matter integrity and cognition in chronic traumatic brain injury: a diffusion tensor imaging study. Brain 2007;130: 2508–19.

50. Johansen-Berg H, Rushworth MFS. Using diffusion imaging to study human connectional anatomy. Annu Rev Neurosci 2009;32:75–94.

51. Schmierer K, Wheeler-Kingshott CA, Boulby PA, et al. Diffusion tensor imaging of post mortem multiple sclerosis brain. Neuroimage 2007;35:467–77.

52. Song S-K, Sun SW, Ramsbottom MJ, et al. Dysmyelination revealed through MRI as increased radial (but unchanged axial) diffusion of water. Neuroimage 2002; 17:1429–36.

53. Song S-K, Yoshino J, Le TQ, et al. Demyelination increases radial diffusivity in corpus callosum of mouse brain. Neuroimage 2005;26:132–40.

54. Wortzel HS, Kraus MF, Filley CM, et al. Diffusion tensor imaging in mild traumatic brain injury litigation. J Am Acad Psychiatry Law 2011;39:511–23.

55. Henry LC, Tremblay J, Tremblay S, et al. Acute and chronic changes in diffusivity measures after sports concussion. J Neurotrauma 2011;28:2049–59.

56. Zhang K, Johnson B, Pennell D, et al. Are functional deficits in concussed individuals consistent with white matter structural alterations: combined FMRI & DTI study. Exp Brain Res 2010;204:57–70.

57. Messé A, Caplain S, Paradot G, et al. Diffusion tensor imaging and white matter lesions at the subacute stage in mild traumatic brain injury with persistent neurobehavioral impairment. Hum Brain Mapp 2011;32:999–1011.

58. McAllister TW, Ford JC, Ji S, et al. Maximum principal strain and strain rate associated with concussion diagnosis correlates with changes in corpus callosum white matter indices. Ann Biomed Eng 2011;40:127–40.

59. Koerte IK, Kaufmann D, Hartl E, et al. A prospective study of physician-observed concussion during a varsity university hockey season: white matter integrity in ice hockey players. Part 3 of 4. Neurosurg Focus 2012;33:E3.

60. Lipton ML, Kim N, Zimmerman ME, et al. Soccer heading is associated with white matter microstructural and cognitive abnormalities. Radiology 2013;268: 850–7.

61. Koerte IK, Ertl-Wagner B, Reiser M, et al. White matter integrity in the brains of professional soccer players without a symptomatic concussion. JAMA 2012; 308:1859–61.

62. Bazarian JJ, Zhong J, Blyth B, et al. Diffusion tensor imaging detects clinically important axonal damage after mild traumatic brain injury: a pilot study. J Neurotrauma 2007;24:1447–59.

63. Bazarian JJ, Zhu T, Blyth B, et al. Subject-specific changes in brain white matter on diffusion tensor imaging after sports-related concussion. Magn Reson Imaging 2012;30:171–80.

64. Cubon VA, Putukian M, Boyer C, et al. A diffusion tensor imaging study on the white matter skeleton in individuals with sports-related concussion. J Neurotrauma 2010;28:189–201.

65. Kumar R, Gupta RK, Husain M, et al. Comparative evaluation of corpus callosum DTI metrics in acute mild and moderate traumatic brain injury: its correlation with neuropsychometric tests. Brain Inj 2009;23:675–85.

66. Lange RT, Iverson GL, Brubacher JR, et al. Diffusion tensor imaging findings are not strongly associated with postconcussional disorder 2 months following mild traumatic brain injury. J Head Trauma Rehabil 2012;27:188–98.

67. Ling JM, Peña A, Yeo RA, et al. Biomarkers of increased diffusion anisotropy in semi-acute mild traumatic brain injury: a longitudinal perspective. Brain 2012; 135:1281–92.

68. Niogi SN, Mukherjee P, Ghajar J, et al. Structural dissociation of attentional control and memory in adults with and without mild traumatic brain injury. Brain 2008;131:3209–21.

69. Niogi SN, Mukherjee P, Ghajar J, et al. Extent of microstructural white matter injury in postconcussive syndrome correlates with impaired cognitive reaction time: a 3T diffusion tensor imaging study of mild traumatic brain injury. AJR Am J Neuroradiol 2008;29:967–73.

70. Borich M, Makan N, Boyd L, et al. Combining whole-brain voxel-wise analysis with in vivo tractography of diffusion behavior after sports-related concussion in adolescents: a preliminary report. J Neurotrauma 2013;30:1243–9.

71. Lingsma HF, Yue JK, Maas AI, et al. Outcome prediction after mild and complicated mild traumatic brain injury: external validation of existing models and identification of new predictors using the TRACK-TBI pilot study. J Neurotrauma 2014;32:83–94.

72. Luther N, Niogi S, Kutner K, et al. Diffusion tensor and susceptibility-weighted imaging in concussion assessment of national football league players. Br J Sports Med 2013;47:e1.

73. Yuh EL, Cooper SR, Mukherjee P, et al. Diffusion tensor imaging for outcome prediction in mild traumatic brain injury: a TRACK-TBI study. J Neurotrauma 2014;31:1457–77.

74. Stippich C. Clinical functional MRI: presurgical functional neuroimaging. Springer - Verlag Berlin Heidelberg; 2015.

75. Fox MD, Greicius M. Clinical applications of resting state functional connectivity. Front Syst Neurosci 2010;4:19.

76. Chen J-K, Johnston KM, Frey S, et al. Functional abnormalities in symptomatic concussed athletes: an fMRI study. Neuroimage 2004;22:68–82.

77. Chen J-K, Johnston KM, Petrides M, et al. Recovery from mild head injury in sports: evidence from serial functional magnetic resonance imaging studies in male athletes. Clin J Sport Med 2008;18:241–7.
78. Dettwiler A, Murugavel M, Putukian M, et al. Persistent differences in patterns of brain activation after sports-related concussion: a longitudinal functional magnetic resonance imaging study. J Neurotrauma 2014;31:180–8.
79. Murugavel M, Cubon V, Putukian M, et al. A Longitudinal Diffusion Tensor Imaging Study Assessing White Matter Fiber Tracts after Sports-Related Concussion. Journal of Neurotrauma 2014;31(22):1860–71.
80. Saluja RS, Chen J-K, Gagnon IJ, et al. Navigational memory functional magnetic resonance imaging: a test for concussion in children. J Neurotrauma 2014;32:712–22.
81. Talavage TM, Nauman EA, Breedlove EL, et al. Functionally-detected cognitive impairment in high school football players without clinically-diagnosed concussion. J Neurotrauma 2010;31:327–38.
82. McAllister TW, Flashman LA, McDonald BC, et al. Mechanisms of working memory dysfunction after mild and moderate TBI: evidence from functional MRI and neurogenetics. J Neurotrauma 2006;23:1450–67.
83. McAllister TW, Sparling MB, Flashman LA, et al. Differential working memory load effects after mild traumatic brain injury. Neuroimage 2001;14:1004–12.
84. Keightley ML, Saluja RS, Chen JK, et al. A functional magnetic resonance imaging study of working memory in youth after sports-related concussion: is it still working? J Neurotrauma 2013;31:437–51.
85. Zhou Y, Milham MP, Lui YW, et al. Default-mode network disruption in mild traumatic brain injury. Radiology 2012;265:882–92.
86. Sours C, Zhuo J, Janowich J, et al. Default mode network interference in mild traumatic brain injury–a pilot resting state study. Brain Res 2013;1537:201–15.
87. Mayer AR, Mannell MV, Ling J, et al. Functional connectivity in mild traumatic brain injury. Hum Brain Mapp 2011;32:1825–35.
88. Johnson B, Zhang K, Gay M, et al. Alteration of brain default network in subacute phase of injury in concussed individuals: resting-state fMRI study. Neuroimage 2012;59:511–8.
89. Stevens MC, Lovejoy D, Kim J, et al. Multiple resting state network functional connectivity abnormalities in mild traumatic brain injury. Brain Imaging Behav 2012;6:293–318.
90. Wintermark M, Sanelli PC, Anzai Y, et al. Imaging evidence and recommendations for traumatic brain injury: conventional neuroimaging techniques. J Am Coll Radiol 2015;12:e1–14.
91. Wintermark M, van Melle G, Schnyder P, et al. Admission perfusion CT: prognostic value in patients with severe head trauma. Radiology 2004;232:211–20.
92. Soustiel JF, Mahamid E, Goldsher D, et al. Perfusion-CT for early assessment of traumatic cerebral contusions. Neuroradiology 2008;50:189–96.
93. Metting Z, Rödiger LA, Stewart RE, et al. Perfusion computed tomography in the acute phase of mild head injury: regional dysfunction and prognostic value. Ann Neurol 2009;66:809–16.
94. Warmuth C, Günther M, Zimmer C. Quantification of blood flow in brain tumors: comparison of arterial spin labeling and dynamic susceptibility-weighted contrast-enhanced MR Imaging. Radiology 2003;228:523–32.
95. Liu W, Wang B, Wolfowitz R, et al. Perfusion deficits in patients with mild traumatic brain injury characterized by dynamic susceptibility contrast MRI. NMR Biomed 2013;26(6):651–63.

96. Ge Y, Patel MB, Chen Q, et al. Assessment of thalamic perfusion in patients with mild traumatic brain injury by true FISP arterial spin labelling MR imaging at 3T. Brain Inj 2009;23:666–74.

97. Wang Y, West JD, Bailey JN, et al. Decreased cerebral blood flow in chronic pediatric mild TBI: an MRI perfusion study. Dev Neuropsychol 2015;40:40–4.

98. Raji CA, Tarzwell R, Pavel D, et al. Clinical utility of SPECT neuroimaging in the diagnosis and treatment of traumatic brain injury: a systematic review. PLoS One 2014;9:e91088.

99. Jacobs A, Put E, Ingels M, et al. Prospective evaluation of Technetium-99m-HMPAO SPECT in mild and moderate traumatic brain injury. J Nucl Med 1994; 35:942–7.

100. Jacobs A, Put E, Ingels M, et al. One-year follow-up of Technetium-99m-HMPAO SPECT in mild head injury. J Nucl Med 1996;37:1605–9.

101. Byrnes KR, Wilson CM, Brabazon F, et al. FDG-PET imaging in mild traumatic brain injury: a critical review. Front Neuroenergetics 2014;5:13.

102. Lin AP, Liao HJ, Merugumala SK, et al. Metabolic imaging of mild traumatic brain injury. Brain Imaging Behav 2012;6:208–23.

103. Stein TD, Alvarez VE, McKee AC. Chronic traumatic encephalopathy: a spectrum of neuropathological changes following repetitive brain trauma in athletes and military personnel. Alzheimers Res Ther 2014;6:4.

104. Barrio JR, Small GW, Wong KP, et al. In vivo characterization of chronic traumatic encephalopathy using [F-18]FDDNP PET brain imaging. Proc Natl Acad Sci U S A 2015;112:E2039–47.

105. Fodero-Tavoletti MT, Okamura N, Furumoto S, et al. 18F-THK523: a novel in vivo tau imaging ligand for Alzheimer's disease. Brain 2011;134:1089–100.

106. Henry LC, Tremblay S, Boulanger Y, et al. Neurometabolic Changes in the acute phase after sports concussions correlate with symptom severity. J Neurotrauma 2009;27:65–76.

107. Sivák Š, Bittšanský M, Grossmann J, et al. Clinical correlations of proton magnetic resonance spectroscopy findings in acute phase after mild traumatic brain injury. Brain Inj 2014;28:341–6.

108. Poole VN, Abbas K, Shenk TE, et al. MR spectroscopic evidence of brain injury in the non-diagnosed collision sport athlete. Dev Neuropsychol 2014;39:459–73.

109. Vagnozzi R, Signoretti S, Cristofori L, et al. Assessment of metabolic brain damage and recovery following mild traumatic brain injury: a multicentre, proton magnetic resonance spectroscopic study in concussed patients. Brain 2010; 133:3232–42.

110. Vagnozzi R, Signoretti S, Tavazzi B, et al. Temporal window of metabolic brain vulnerability to concussion: a pilot 1H-magnetic resonance spectroscopic study in concussed athletes–part III. Neurosurgery 2008;62:1286–95 [discussion: 1295–6].

111. Vagnozzi R, Signoretti S, Floris R, et al. Decrease in N-acetylaspartate following concussion may be coupled to decrease in creatine. J Head Trauma Rehabil 2013;28:284–92.

112. Henry LC, Tremblay S, Leclerc S, et al. Metabolic changes in concussed American football players during the acute and chronic post-injury phases. BMC Neurol 2011;11:105.

Returning to School Following Sport-Related Concussion

Grant L. Iverson, PhD[a,b,c,d,e], Gerard A. Gioia, PhD[f],*

KEYWORDS

- Sports • Concussion • Mild traumatic brain injury • TBI • Youth • Pediatric

KEY POINTS

- There are individual differences in how and when to return to school following sport-related concussion. Some return immediately and fully, and others benefit from a gradual approach. A supportive and progressive approach to the return to school is recommended.
- A key principle for youth with symptoms persisting beyond the first week is to learn how to engage in optimal activity levels (ie, maximizing activity and productivity while minimizing exacerbation of symptoms).
- Individualized, targeted accommodations can be helpful to facilitate a faster, less stressful, and successful return to school.

INTRODUCTION

Following sport-related concussion, the first priority for children and adolescents is the safe, swift, effective, and sustained return to school. The second priority is a full and successful return to extracurricular activities—including sports. Consensus-based practice recommendations emphasize that student athletes should rest following

Declaration of Conflicting Interests: See last page of article.

Funding: G. Gioia notes that this article was supported in part by CDC Awards U17/CCU323352 and U49CE001385, and NIH Grants #M01RR020359 from the National Center for Research Resources (NCRR), a component of the National Institutes of Health (NIH), and NIH #P30/HDO40677-07.

[a] Department of Physical Medicine and Rehabilitation, Harvard Medical School, Boston, MA, USA; [b] Spaulding Rehabilitation Hospital, Boston, MA, USA; [c] MassGeneral Hospital for Children Sport Concussion Program, Boston, MA, USA; [d] Home Base Program, Red Sox Foundation, Massachusetts General Hospital, Boston, MA, USA; [e] Department of Physical Medicine and Rehabilitation, Center for Health and Rehabilitation, Harvard Medical School, 79/96 Thirteenth Street, Charlestown Navy Yard, Charlestown, MA 02129, USA; [f] Department of Pediatrics and Psychiatry & Behavioral Sciences, Division of Pediatric Neuropsychology, Children's National Health System, George Washington University School of Medicine, 15245 Shady Grove Road, Suite 350, Rockville, MD 20850, USA
* Corresponding author.
E-mail address: ggioia@childrensnational.org

Phys Med Rehabil Clin N Am 27 (2016) 429–436
http://dx.doi.org/10.1016/j.pmr.2015.12.002
1047-9651/16/$ – see front matter © 2016 Elsevier Inc. All rights reserved.

injury, gradually resume activities, and that children should be treated more conservatively than college and professional athletes.[1] The tripartite recommendation for rest, gradual activation, and conservatism presents challenges for the clinician. Specific evidence-based recommendations for how to implement this general management strategy are not available. Nevertheless, practical and logical recommendations can be provided to reintegrate the student back into the school environment, and to provide guidance regarding activities that might provoke or exacerbate symptoms during the day. This process requires a constructive working relationship between the school and the community health care provider who is managing the medical recovery; both bring essential skills to the process.[2] According to meta-analyses of the available literature, sport-related concussions have a large adverse effect on cognition in the first 24 hours with resolution of these deficits occurring within about 1 week, according to group studies.[3,4] Clinicians working with injured athletes, especially high school students, know that many take much longer to recover. In fact, in a prospective study of high school football players, only 42% to 47% were deemed functionally recovered by 1 week (Figure 1, Collins, et al., "Sport-related concussion" in *Brain injury medicine: principles and* practice, 2012, page 503).[5,6] It was not until 4 weeks that 84% to 94% were considered recovered. Clearly, sport-related concussion causes symptoms (eg, headaches and fatigue) and cognitive difficulties that can make it difficult for a student to be effective in school.

To define the types of school-related problems experienced by students, a clinic sample of elementary, middle, and high school students (n = 216) was asked to describe postinjury problems that they were having in school.[7] They reported difficulty paying attention (58%), understanding new material (44%), and slowed performance when completing homework (49%). In addition, they reported headaches interfering with learning (66%) and fatigue in class (54%). High school students reported more of these in-school problems than students in younger grade levels. The number of school problems was positively correlated with postconcussion symptoms,[7] indicating that the more symptomatic students tended to struggle the most in school.

This article addresses a gap in the published literature. The foundation for this article is an article by Gioia[2] and materials from the Center for Disease Control and Prevention concussion education program.[8] The reader can also obtain educational materials from 3 other sources for school management and supports: the Colorado Reduce, Educate, Adjust/Accommodate, Pace (REAP) program,[9] the Oregon Brain 101 program,[10] and Pennsylvania's BrainSTEPS program.[11] At a systems level, Gioia and colleagues[12] have articulated the essential components of an educational infrastructure to support the return to school of students following concussion. Ideally, state and local policies for return to school are in place to promote implementation of a consistent process. The 5 components to build this support infrastructure include: (1) defining and training an interdisciplinary school concussion management team, (2) professional development of the school and medical communities with respect to concussion management in the school; (3) identification, assessment, and progress monitoring protocols; (4) availability of a flexible set of intervention strategies to accommodate the student's recovery needs; and (5) systematized protocols for active communication among medical, school, and family team members.

School personnel and health care providers play important and cooperative roles in the provision of supports for the returning student with a concussion. School personnel provide their expertise in developing the academic accommodations and adjustments; however, they need guidance from the health care provider on the specific targets toward which they should direct the school supports. The medical evaluation and the resulting student symptom profile is the first step to constructing the plan of accommodations and adjustments. An assessment using a standardized questionnaire can define the key symptom targets that the school can address in their intervention plan. In addition, the health care provider can work with the student and parent, using basic education and reassurance about a positive recovery, providing general guidance regarding activity allowances and restrictions, and discussing the types of targeted strategies available to manage and alleviate specific symptoms.

RECOMMENDATIONS FOR RETURN TO SCHOOL FOLLOWING INJURY

There are considerable individual differences in the rate at which students are ready to return to school following injury, with some returning immediately and fully and others returning gradually with accommodations. The authors typically encourage youth to return to school during the first week following injury and, if symptomatic, we encourage accommodations. Those who have not returned in 2 weeks should be evaluated carefully to determine why because prolonged absence from school can have significant negative effects. Several different accommodations might be reasonable and necessary during the initial days, and sometimes weeks, following injury. Examples of these accommodations are provided in **Table 1**. As previously noted, the health care provider's initial evaluation of symptoms is a good place to start in developing the accommodations plan. **Table 1** provides examples of how symptoms cause challenges in school, with various accommodations that can be used to reduce symptoms and improve overall functioning in school. Some students might benefit from a small number of accommodations for only a few days, whereas students with symptoms that persist for several weeks might benefit from more accommodations and a careful management plan to facilitate their academic success. Regular monitoring of symptoms with adjustments to the accommodations as the student progresses through recovery can be helpful.

Gioia[2] proposed a model for assisting children and adolescents with returning to school following injury. This model has 6 stages (**Table 2**). This model is designed as a general framework for clinicians; it is meant to be tailored to the individualized needs of the patient. The rate at which a person progresses through the stages varies, and some students can skip certain stages. This model, combined with some accommodations from **Table 1** and progressive activity engagement (**Table 3**), can be very helpful for youth who struggle with symptoms that are interfering with their academics.

The Progressive Activities of Controlled Exertion (PACE) approach,[2] presented in **Table 3**, is organized into 4 stages. During the first stage, the clinician (1) establishes a positive, optimistic, active problem-solving context (ie, "We can solve this recovery problem."); (2) evaluates the youth's emotional response to injury (ie, "This is how I am feeling and it helps or hinders me in my recovery."); and (3) provides education and reassurance (ie, "With your knowledge of concussion and controlling your activity level, you will get better."). In the second stage, the clinician (1) works with the youth and parents to define a daily schedule, (2) learns about the associations between certain activities and symptom exacerbation, and (3) better understands what activities lead to the greatest symptoms so those can be targeted for monitoring and modification. In the third stage, the clinician teaches important concepts such as (1) engaging in "not too little and not too much" activity, (2) engaging in "reasonable" symptom monitoring (being careful to not reinforce anxious monitoring, hypervigilance, or catastrophizing), and (3) pacing oneself so that the student can be productive

Table 1
Postconcussion symptoms and functional school problems as targets for academic accommodations

Postconcussion Symptoms	Functional School Problem	Accommodation or Management Strategy
Attention or Concentration	Short focus on lecture, classwork, homework	Shorter assignments, break down tasks, lighter work load
Working Memory	Holding instructions in mind, reading comprehension, math calculation, writing	Repetition, written instructions, use of calculator, short reading passages
Memory Consolidation or Retrieval	Retaining new information, accessing learned info when needed	Smaller amounts to learn, recognition cues
Processing Speed	Keep pace with work demand, process verbal information effectively	Extended time, slow down verbal info, comprehension-checking
Cognitive Fatigue	Decreased arousal or activation to engage basic attention, working memory	Rest breaks during classes, homework, and examinations
Anxiety	Interferes with concentration; student may push through symptoms to prevent falling behind	Reassurance from teachers and team about accommodations; workload reduction, alternate forms of testing
Depression or Withdrawal	Withdrawal from school or friends due to stigma or activity restrictions	Engage student with friends at lunch or recess, build in time for socialization
Irritability	Poor tolerance for stress, alienate peers or teachers	Reduce stimulation and stressors, provide rest break
Headaches	Interferes with concentration, increased irritability	Rest breaks, short nap
Light or Noise Sensitivity	Symptoms worsen in bright or loud environments	Temporarily wear sunglasses, seating away from bright sunlight or other light; avoid noisy or crowded environments such as lunchroom, assemblies, and hallways
Dizziness or Balance Problems	Unsteadiness when walking	Elevator pass, class transition before bell
Sleep Disturbance	Decreased arousal, shifted sleep schedule	Later start time, shortened day
Symptom Sensitivity (exertional effects)	Symptoms worsen with over-activity, resulting in any of the previously listed problems	Reduce cognitive or physical demands below symptom threshold; provide rest breaks; complete work in small increments until symptom threshold increases

Adapted from Gioia GA. Medical-school partnership in guiding return to school following mild traumatic brain injury in youth. J Child Neurol 2014;31(1):100.

but not push too hard resulting in a significant exacerbation of symptoms. During the fourth stage, the clinician (1) emphasizes the dynamic nature of the recovery process, (2) that exertion-related symptoms might vary during this process, and that (3) gradually building the capacity and tolerance for activities is preferred.

Table 2
Gradual return to academics

Stage	Description	Activity Level	Criteria to Move to Next Stage
0	No return, at home	Maintain low level cognitive and physical activity; no prolonged concentration Cognitive readiness challenge: as symptoms improve, try reading or math challenge task for 10–30 minutes; assess for symptom increase	1. Student can sustain concentration for 30 minutes before significant symptom exacerbation 2. Symptoms reduce or disappear with cognitive rest breaks,[a] allowing the student to return to the activity
1	Return to school, partial day (1–3 hours)	Attend 1–3 classes, with interspersed rest breaks; minimal expectations for productivity; no tests or homework	Student's symptoms are improving, able to tolerate 4–5 hours of activity with 2–3 cognitive rest breaks built into school day
2	Full day, maximal supports (maximal supports needed throughout day)	Attend most classes, with 2–3 rest breaks (20–30 minutes), no tests; minimal homework ($\leq$60 minutes); minimal-moderate expectations for productivity	Number and severity of symptoms improving, and needs only 1–2 cognitive rest breaks built into school day
3	Full day, moderate supports (moderate supports provided in response to symptoms during the day)	Attend all classes with 1–2 rest breaks (20–30 minutes); begin quizzes; moderate homework (60–90 minutes); moderate expectations for productivity; design schedule for make-up work	Continued symptom improvement, and needs no more than 1 cognitive rest break per day
4	Full day, minimal supports (monitoring final recovery)	Attend all classes with 0–1 rest breaks (20–30 minutes); begin modified tests (with breaks and/or extra time, if needed); normal homework schedule (90 + minutes); moderate-maximum expectations for productivity	No active symptoms throughout the school day
5	Full return, no supports needed	Full class schedule, no rest breaks; maximum expectations for productivity; begin to address make-up work	—

[a] A period during which the student refrains from academic or other cognitively demanding activities, including schoolwork, reading, television, or games, and conversation. This can involve a short nap or relaxation with eyes closed in a quiet setting.

Adapted from Gioia GA. Medical-school partnership in guiding return to school following mild traumatic brain injury in youth. J Child Neurol 2014;31(1):98.

Table 3
Concussion activity-exertion management: progressive activities of controlled exertion

Stage	Treatment Component	Description
Set the Positive Foundation	1. Establish a positive, active problem-solving context	Provide the student, family, and school with a psychologically positive, active problem-solving context for rehabilitation. Framing the injury and its recovery in a positive, progressive, reassuring manner is critical.
	2. Assess and manage emotional response to injury	Explore the emotional response of the child and family to the injury. Assess how it has disrupted their lives. Ask what stresses or demands they are facing (school, peer, athletics).
	3. Developmentally appropriate education about mTBI and its effects	Provide developmentally appropriate education regarding the dynamics of mTBI (ie, software injury, energy deficit), and the relationship between the student's level of activity and symptom exacerbation (exertional effects). Review the sources of exertion: physical, cognitive, emotional, and the need to manage these energy demands.
Define the Parameters of Activity-Exertion	4a. Define daily schedule	a. Define the student's typical daily schedule (before, during, after school, weekends)
	4b. Define type, intensity, and duration of cognitive and physical activities, and their exertional effects	b. Define times of the day when activities present the greatest exertional challenges ("hot spots") and lesser challenges ("cool spots"). Identify the type, intensity, and duration of cognitive and physical activities within the daily schedule.
	5. Define tolerability for activity intensity and duration	Define limits of tolerability for activity intensity or duration. Identify when symptoms do not increase substantially. This should be done for each key class. Sample question: "How long can you typically go in your classes before you notice your symptoms worsening and affecting your learning?" Use time or intensity limits to schedule "work-rest" breaks.
Teach Activity-Exertion Monitoring	6. Teach "Not too little, not too much" concept	Teach the concept of moderated activity (ie, engaging in "Not too little, but not too much" activity). The student's goal is to find the activity "sweet spot" in whichactivity time and effort are maximized without symptoms worsening.
	7. Teach reasonable symptom monitoring	Teach "reasonable" symptom monitoring and recording. Be aware of child or parent that is, overly anxious or oblivious. Coach them to monitor symptoms reasonably.
	8. Teach working to tolerable limits using a work-rest-work-rest approach	Instruct the student to work up to their symptom limits but to not exceed them, by being aware of (ie, reasonable monitoring) their symptoms. Emphasize tolerance of a mild increase in symptoms, but not excessive increase.

(continued on next page)

Table 3 (continued)		
Stage	**Treatment Component**	**Description**
Reinforce Progress	9. Recovery is dynamic; activity-exertion management will reduce symptoms	Instruct that the recovery process is dynamic, controlled activity-exertion management will feel better, and symptoms will decrease. Highlight examples of resolving symptoms as evidence of progress toward recovery.
	10. Gradual increase activity time or intensity.	As symptoms reduce with greater tolerance for activity, gradually increase the time or intensity of activity. The "sweet spot" of activity-exertion will move closer to their norm.

Abbreviation: mTBI, mild traumatic brain injury.
Adapted from Gioia GA. Medical-school partnership in guiding return to school following mild traumatic brain injury in youth. J Child Neurol 2014;31(1):101.

The whole approach previously discussed and illustrated in **Tables 1–3** is meant to be adapted and tailored to the specific needs of the student. Movement through the plan should be systematic and at a pace that makes clinical sense. A positive, collaborative, problem-solving approach between the clinician, family, and school increases the probability of success in difficult cases.

SUMMARY

Returning to school following concussion can go smoothly and uneventfully, or it can be difficult. Very little published research is available to assist clinicians with helping student athletes swiftly and effectively return to school following injury. Clinicians can provide practical and logical guidance for using academic accommodations to manage symptoms during the school day. The return to school process is best facilitated by an established relationship between defined school personnel (eg, school nurse, athletic trainer) and the community health care provider, each with their own roles and responsibilities in the support of the student. Research is needed to examine the efficacy and efficiency of this staged approach to returning to school, and the specific recommendations for managing activity level and symptom response during this process. Moving forward, more user-friendly clinician materials and handouts need to be developed to facilitate the process of educating and guiding injured students, families, and school personnel. It also would be helpful to develop a manualized approach to delivering this service, and then evaluating its time-effectiveness, cost-effectiveness, and usefulness.

DECLARATION OF CONFLICTING INTERESTS

G. Gioia is a test coauthor of the Behavior Rating Inventory of Executive Function for which he receives royalties. He is a coauthor of the Acute Concussion Evaluation (ACE), ACE Care Plan, and ACE Home/School Instructions, for which he receives no remuneration. G.L. Iverson has been reimbursed by the government, professional scientific bodies, and commercial organizations for discussing or presenting research relating to mild traumatic brain injury (TBI) and sport-related concussion at meetings, scientific conferences, and symposiums. He has a clinical practice in forensic neuropsychology involving individuals who have sustained mild TBIs (including athletes). He has received honorariums for serving on research panels that provide scientific peer review of programs. He is a coinvestigator, collaborator, or consultant on grants funded by several organizations relating to mild TBI.

ACKNOWLEDGMENTS

G.L. Iverson acknowledges support from the Mooney-Reed Charitable Foundation.

REFERENCES

1. McCrory P, Meeuwisse WH, Aubry M, et al. Consensus statement on concussion in sport: the 4th International Conference on Concussion in Sport held in Zurich, November 2012. Br J Sports Med 2013;47:250–8.
2. Gioia GA. Medical-school partnership in guiding return to school following mild traumatic brain injury in youth. J Child Neurol 2016;31(1):93–108.
3. Broglio SP, Puetz TW. The effect of sport concussion on neurocognitive function, self-report symptoms and postural control: a meta-analysis. Sports Med 2008;38: 53–67.
4. Belanger HG, Vanderploeg RD. The neuropsychological impact of sports-related concussion: a meta-analysis. J Int Neuropsychol Soc 2005;11:345–57.
5. Collins MW, Lovell MR, Iverson GL, et al. Examining concussion rates and return to play in high school football players wearing newer helmet technology: a three year prospective cohort study. Neurosurgery 2006;58:275–86.
6. Collins MW, Iverson GL, Gaetz M, et al. Sport-related concussion. In: Zasler ND, Katz DI, Zafonte RD, editors. Brain injury medicine: principles and practice. 2nd edition. New York: Demos Medical Publishing; 2012. p. 498–516.
7. Sady MD, Vaughan CG, Gioia GA. School and the concussed youth: recommendations for concussion education and management. Phys Med Rehabil Clin N Am 2011;22:701–19, ix.
8. Centers for Disease Control and Prevention. Heads up to schools: know your concussion ABCs. 2015. Available at: http://www.cdc.gov/concussion/HeadsUp/schools.html. Accessed November 19, 2015.
9. Rocky Mountain Hospital for Children. Concussion management/REAP 2015. Available at: http://rockymountainhospitalforchildren.com/service/concussion-management-reap-guidelines. Accessed November 19, 2015.
10. Brain 101: The Concussion Playbook. School-wide concussion management. 2011. Available at: http://brain101.orcasinc.com/. Accessed November 19, 2015.
11. Pennsylvania Department of Education, Brain Injury Association of Pennsylvania, Pennsylvania Department of Health. BrainSTEPS: strategies teaching educators, parents, and students. Available at: www.brainsteps.net. Accessed November 19, 2015.
12. Gioia GA, Glang A, Hooper S, et al. Building statewide infrastructure for the academic support of students with mild traumatic brain injury. J Head Trauma Rehabil 2015. [Epub ahead of print].

Active Rehabilitation of Concussion and Post-concussion Syndrome

John J. Leddy, MD[a],*, John G. Baker, PhD[b], Barry Willer, PhD[c]

KEYWORDS

- Rehabilitation • Concussion • Post-concussion syndrome • Active
- Physiology • Treatment

KEY POINTS

- Patients with concussion are advised to rest until all symptoms resolve. Recent research suggests that a more active approach to concussion management may be beneficial.
- Practitioners should perform a physical examination in patients with concussion and PCS to try to identify one or more potentially treatable post-concussion disorders.
- Active treatments (e.g., subthreshold aerobic exercise and/or cervical, vestibular, cognitive behavioral, and vision therapy) may improve recovery from concussion if implemented at the right time.

INTRODUCTION

Rest has been the mainstay of the treatment for concussion.[1] Research based on animal physiological concussion studies suggests that the concussed human brain is in a vulnerable state that places it at increased risk of more debilitating injury should it sustain more trauma or experience undue stress before metabolic homeostasis has been restored.[2,3] This vulnerable state can be inferred to exist in humans after concussion from the rare but devastating (and controversial) phenomenon of second impact syndrome,[4,5] from data that concussion risk increases after having had one or more concussions[6] and from retrospective data suggesting that high levels of physical and/or cognitive activity soon after concussion delay recovery.[7] The timing and amount of rest after concussion have not been established; as such, the most recent world consensus concussion statement recommends that an initial period of rest in the acute symptomatic period following injury (24–48 hours) may be beneficial, followed by gradual return to school and social activities (before contact sports) in a manner

[a] UBMD Department of Orthopaedics and Sports Medicine, SUNY Buffalo, 160 Farber Hall, Buffalo, NY 14214, USA; [b] UBMD Department of Orthopaedics and Sports Medicine and Nuclear Medicine, Jacobs School of Medicine and Biomedical Sciences, School of Social Work, University at Buffalo, Buffalo, NY, USA; [c] Department of Psychiatry, Jacobs School of Medicine and Biomedical Sciences, University at Buffalo, Buffalo, NY, USA
* Corresponding author.
E-mail address: leddy@buffalo.edu

Phys Med Rehabil Clin N Am 27 (2016) 437–454
http://dx.doi.org/10.1016/j.pmr.2015.12.003
1047-9651/16/$ – see front matter © 2016 Elsevier Inc. All rights reserved.

that does not result in a significant exacerbation of symptoms.[8] The concept of "rest until asymptomatic" is also recommended by some clinicians when advising patients with prolonged recovery after concussion, which is called post-concussion syndrome (PCS).[1,9] Recent clinical and experimental studies are, however, beginning to challenge the utility of prolonged rest as treatment of concussion and PCS.[1,10] The purpose of this article is to review the emerging evidence for the active, nonpharmacologic rehabilitation of concussion and PCS.

DEFINITION OF CONCUSSION

- Concussion is a brain injury that involves a complex pathophysiological process induced by biomechanical forces.[8]
- This complex pathophysiological process includes metabolic,[2] physiological,[11] and microstructural[12] injury to the brain that produces excitatory neurotransmitter release, abnormal ion fluxes, increased glucose metabolism, lactic acid accumulation, and inflammation.
- The macrophysiological insult to the brain affects the autonomic nervous system (ANS) and its control of both cerebral blood flow (CBF) and cardiac rhythm.[13]
- The majority (80%–90%) of sport-related concussions (SRC) in adults resolve in a short (7–10 days) period, although the recovery time frame may be longer in children and adolescents.[8]
- Recent research that accounts for vestibular-oculomotor problems that often accompany SRC suggests that recovery time for adolescents after SRC may take 3 to 4 weeks, which is longer than the commonly reported 7 to 14 days.[14]

DEFINITION OF POST-CONCUSSION SYNDROME

In some cases, concussion symptoms are prolonged.[8] Persistence of symptoms beyond the generally accepted time frame for recovery is called "post-concussion syndrome."

- PCS is not a single pathophysiological entity. It is a term used to describe a constellation of nonspecific symptoms (eg, headache, fatigue, sleep disturbance, vertigo, irritability, anxiety, depression, apathy, and difficulty with concentration and exercise) that are linked to several possible causes that do not necessarily reflect ongoing physiological brain injury.[9]
- The differential diagnosis of PCS includes depression, somatization, chronic fatigue, chronic pain, cervical injury, vestibular dysfunction, ocular dysfunction, or some combination of these conditions.[15]
- The challenge for clinicians is to determine whether prolonged symptoms after concussion reflect a prolonged version of the concussion pathophysiology versus a manifestation of a secondary process such as premorbid clinical depression, a cervical injury, or migraine headaches.[16,17] It is therefore essential that the clinician obtain a history of prior affective or medical problems, perform a careful physical examination, and consider the response to exertion (ie, whether exertion reliably exacerbates symptoms)[18] when developing the differential diagnosis of persistent post-concussion symptoms. Through this process, the clinician may be able to link symptoms of post-concussion "syndrome" to one or more definable post-concussion "disorders."[19] For example, establishing a premorbid history of migraine headaches, depression, anxiety, attention deficit hyperactivity disorder, or learning disability is crucial because concussion can exacerbate these conditions, and they in turn can be responsible for ongoing symptoms.[17]

The accepted time frame for recovery after concussion is not scientifically established and depends on the circumstances of the clinical scenario.

- Persistent symptoms (>10 days) are, for example, generally reported in 10% to 15% of SRC.[8]
- In patients with non-SRC, however, PCS is defined as symptoms persisting for more than 3 months.[20,21]
- Some studies have identified risk factors for persistent symptoms, such as age (younger), sex (female), and history of (multiple) prior concussions.[6,22,23]
- The Zurich Consensus Guidelines state that, in general, symptoms are not specific to concussion, and it is important to consider other abnormalities.[8] This statement was confirmed in a recent study of patients with persistent symptoms for more than 3 weeks after head injury, which included cognitive symptoms that traditionally have been ascribed to brain injury. In this study, cognitive, somatic, and behavioral symptoms did not reliably discriminate between patients with physiological post-concussion disorder (defined as those with persisting symptoms who demonstrated exercise intolerance on a treadmill test) from patients with cervicogenic and/or vestibular post-concussion disorders (defined as those with persisting symptoms who had normal exercise tolerance but abnormal cervical and/or vestibular physical examinations).[19]

NONPHARMACOLOGIC TREATMENT APPROACHES
Acute Concussion

Rest

- The most recent Zurich Consensus statement on concussion in sport recommends that patients should rest for 24 to 48 hours after concussion.[8] This recommendation is reasonable because symptoms can increase with cognitive and physical exertion shortly after concussion.[7,24]
- Rest is also one of the most common recommendations patients who sustain non-SRC receive following head trauma.[25] There are experimental human data to support this recommendation. Functional MRI (fMRI) studies in those performing cognitive tasks have reported that excessive (compensatory) brain activation (as measured by fMRI blood flow) is a feature of concussion, suggesting that the brain should be rested after concussion because the threshold for physical exertion may also be lowered.[26,27]
- There are emerging data that excessive cognitive activity soon after concussion exacerbates symptoms and may delay recovery.[28]

What remains to be scientifically established, however, is just what "rest" means in the setting of concussion (eg, physical? cognitive? both?) and for how long it should be prescribed. "Rest" may be interpreted to include anything from strict bedrest to relative rest from intense athletic activity.

- The duration of rest after SRC is generally interpreted to mean "until asymptomatic" (the 2012 Zurich Consensus statement says "The cornerstone of concussion management is physical and cognitive rest until the acute symptoms resolve").[8]
- Symptoms after head injury are not specific to the brain (eg, they can originate from the cervical spine[19]) and healthy, nonconcussed persons report some degree of symptoms on traditional concussion symptom checklists.[29]
- The use of symptom resolution to define an optimally therapeutic amount of rest is therefore fraught with difficulty, and how patients interpret "rest" is

inconsistent. In a prospective study, de Kruijk and colleagues[30] randomized adults discharged from the emergency department (ED) with acute mild traumatic brain injury (mTBI) to usual care or strict bedrest and found no significant differences in actual amounts of reported rest or in outcomes at 2 weeks, 3 months, and 6 months after injury.

It is clear that some rest, both physical and cognitive, is beneficial to allow the brain to recover from the acute metabolic crisis of concussion. Conversely, too much rest after concussion may have adverse physiological and psychological consequences and contribute to prolonged symptoms.

- Abnormal control of CBF appears to be a fundamental physiological disturbance after concussion.[31–33] Physical inactivity negatively affects CBF control,[34] whereas regular physical activity enhances CBF control.[35]
- Exercise intolerance is a sign of ongoing physiological dysregulation after concussion.[36]
- Exercise intolerance as a result of abnormally elevated CBF during physical exertion has been associated with prolonged inactivity in female athletes with persistent symptoms after concussion.[31] In this study, a program of individualized subthreshold aerobic exercise treatment restored the control of CBF to normal in association with return of exercise tolerance and with symptom resolution.

It is generally accepted that children and adolescents require more cognitive and physical rest in the acute phase of concussion recovery, theoretically because of the unique requirements of the developing brain.[8]

- Recent evidence suggests, however, that children may recover faster than adolescents from concussion.[37] This evidence may relate to the widely variable nonlinear trajectories in CBF evolution that have been observed during adolescent development.[38]
- In adults who sustain a concussion, there is no evidence that complete rest beyond 3 days is beneficial to their recovery.[1] In athletes, prolonged rest after concussion can lead to physical deconditioning and secondary symptoms such as fatigue and reactive depression.[39]
- The challenge to clinicians is to use rest to aid in the recovery from the acute effects of concussion but to avoid "rest until asymptomatic" as a long-term prescription for those patients whose symptoms persist for weeks or months.

Return to normal activity

The most recent Zurich Consensus statement on concussion in sport recommends that patients should gradually return to school and social activities in a manner that does not result in a significant exacerbation of symptoms.[8]

- In a prospective study of concussed patients in a pediatric ED, Thomas and colleagues[10] randomly assigned patients aged 11 to 22 years within 24 hours of concussion to strict rest for 5 days versus 1 to 2 days of strict rest followed by stepwise return to regular daily activities. Consistent with their recommendation, the intervention (strict rest) group reported significantly less school and afterschool attendance for days 2 to 5 post-concussion (3.8 vs 6.7 hours total). There were no clinically significant differences in neurocognitive or balance outcomes. Interestingly, however, the strict 5 days rest group reported more daily post-concussive symptoms and slower symptom resolution than the group who rested for 1 to 2 days. The investigators concluded that recommending strict rest for adolescents immediately after concussion offered no added benefit over usual care.

- A recent prospective study evaluated a prescribed day of cognitive and physical rest after concussion. Patients in the rest group were withheld from activities, including classes, for the remainder of the injury day and the following day, whereas patients in the no-rest group were not provided any after-injury accommodations. Prescribed rest did not reduce post-concussion recovery time, suggesting that light activity after concussion may not be deleterious to recovery.[40]
- In a retrospective study of student athletes, those who reported engaging in a medium level of physical and cognitive activity (ie, school activity and light activity at home, such as slow jogging or mowing the lawn) had fewer symptoms and performed better on neurocognitive testing than those who reported engaging in high levels of activity (ie, school activity and sports practice or school activity and participation in a sports game) but also compared with those reporting very low levels of activity (ie, no school or exercise activity or school activity only),[7] suggesting that participation in typical daily activities soon after concussion is associated with better recovery. These findings should be cautiously interpreted because activity was self-reported recall, and it is not known at what point after injury the athletes began physical activity.
- In a prospective study of activity reports after brain injury,[41] just more than 20% of 126 mTBI subjects recruited from an ED reported symptoms consistent with PCS at 3 and 6 months. Negative mTBI perceptions, stress, anxiety, depression, and all-or-nothing behavior were associated with the risk of PCS. Multivariate analysis revealed that all-or-nothing behavior, which was defined as either excessive activity ("pushing through") or complete rest ("crashing") over the first 2 weeks following injury, was the key predictor for the onset of PCS at 3 months after injury. Negative mTBI perceptions best predicted PCS 6 months after injury. The investigators concluded that patients' perceptions of their head injury and their behavioral responses play important roles in the development of PCS.

Post-concussion Syndrome

Rest

The primary forms of PCS treatment have traditionally included a recommendation for rest until symptoms subside along with other interventions, such as education, coping techniques, support and reassurance, neurocognitive rehabilitation, and antidepressants.[42] With respect to rest versus activity, long-term adverse consequences of early activity sufficient to provoke or exacerbate symptoms have been hypothesized in humans because animal studies have shown negative effects of exercise shortly after concussion.

- Griesbach and colleagues[43] reported that premature voluntary exercise within the first week after rodent concussion impaired cognitive performance, whereas aerobic exercise performed 14 to 21 days after concussion improved performance. They also showed that cardiac and temperature autonomic regulation were compromised during exercise within the first 2 weeks after injury.[44]
- In a subsequent study, they analyzed the effects of voluntary versus forced exercise after concussion. Rats *forced* to exercise 28 to 32 days and 35 to 39 days after mTBI markedly stimulated the corticotropic axis and did not increase brain-derived neurotrophic factor (BDNF), which is involved in neuron repair after injury, whereas BDNF levels increased following *voluntary* exercise.[45]

- In another study, rats forced to exercise after mTBI/concussion increased the cortisol/corticotropin stress response, whereas rats allowed to voluntarily exercise did not, suggesting that exercise regimens with strong stress responses (ie, forced exercise) may not be beneficial during the early posttraumatic brain injury (TBI) period.[46] Thus, the motivation and circumstances surrounding exercise appear to be important after mTBI.
- Other animal researchers have identified beneficial effects of early exercise shortly after mTBI on various measures of brain neuroplasticity.[47–50]
- The bulk of the animal data suggests that uncontrolled or forced activity too soon after concussion is detrimental to recovery, but that voluntary exercise is not and may enhance recovery.

Athletes

- Prolonged rest, especially in athletes, can lead to physical deconditioning,[39] metabolic disturbances,[51] and secondary symptoms, such as fatigue and reactive depression.[52]
- As stated above, there are some retrospective human data showing that athletes who reported quite high levels of activity soon after concussion had worse neurocognitive performance than those who reported moderate levels of activity.[7]
- In athletes who remain symptomatic for weeks to months after concussion, it has been shown that symptom-limited exercise testing using a predetermined stopping criterion (symptom exacerbation) is safe and reliable.[53,54] The data are used to prescribe individualized progressive subthreshold aerobic exercise treatment that has been shown to be effective and safe and that can positively affect outcome at 1 year after injury.[18,55]
- Inactivity has been shown to prolong recovery from many health conditions, including those most often comorbid with mTBI/concussion, such as vestibular disorders, depression, posttraumatic stress disorder, chronic fatigue, and pain disorders.[1] It is therefore essential to establish the differential diagnosis of prolonged symptoms after concussion because postconcussion disorders will often respond to active intervention.

Active rehabilitation for post-concussion syndrome

Psychosocial factors and cognitive rehabilitation The empirical support for active psychological and neuropsychological rehabilitation specifically for PCS is somewhat limited.[56] Several recent review articles have noted the importance of addressing concussion knowledge, symptom interpretation, recovery expectations and other thought patterns, and activity levels, in preventing and managing persistent symptoms after concussion.[9,57,58] The potential benefit of integrating cognitive behavioral therapy (CBT) to address thoughts and activities with cognitive rehabilitation to address difficulties with cognitive abilities, such as attention and memory, has also been noted.[59] These approaches to active rehabilitation are grouped into psychoeducational, psychological, and cognitive interventions and reviewed in later discussion. A comprehensive and multidisciplinary approach to treatment, consistent with the concept that PCS can involve more than one disorder, appears promising.

Psychoeducational intervention

- Reassurance, discussing expected recovery time, and educating about compensatory strategies early on can improve symptoms of PCS.[60] Two controlled adult studies have shown that brief, early education (an information booklet)[61] and psychological intervention[62] can reduce PCS symptoms at 3 to 6 months after injury.

- With respect to functional outcome in PCS, there are 3 randomized controlled trials (RCTs) that used education (for example, that problems after injury were common and would probably disappear within a few months), support/reassurance, coping strategies (for example, introduction of structured daily activities and keeping a diary), information sheets on gradual return to normal activities, ongoing advice (over a period of 6–12 months), and regular follow-up visits. Wade and colleagues[63] found that this approach improved daily social functioning and reduced PCS symptoms at 6 months in adults, whereas others found that education and early treatment inadvertently enhanced patients' consciousness of their symptoms and increased disability.[64,65] Thus, results of this form of treatment are mixed.

Psychological intervention

- A systematic review in 2010 of psychological interventions for the treatment of PCS concluded that there was limited evidence so far in the existing literature of benefit from rehabilitation programs with a psychotherapeutic element.[15] This review also discussed CBT, which is a form of psychological intervention that focuses on identifying and changing patterns of maladaptive thinking and behavior that can exacerbate, or in some cases even cause, affective symptoms often associated with persistent effects of direct brain injury, including depression and anxiety. Three RCTs and 7 other studies of CBT all found some benefit, although there were limitations in study design.[9,15] Since that review, a pilot clinical trial with 28 participants at risk for PCS compared treatment as usual (education, reassurance, and symptom management strategies) from an occupational therapist to this treatment plus CBT from a psychologist.[66] Participants at risk for PCS were identified based on a multivariate prediction model that included symptom severity and the beliefs that symptoms will persist and will have catastrophic life consequences.[67] Fewer at-risk participants who received CBT had a diagnosis of PCS at follow-up (54% vs 91%, $P<.05$). Treatment effect sizes were moderate for symptoms (Cohen d = 0.74) and moderate to large for most other secondary outcome measures (Cohen d = 0.62–1.61).
- A recent RCT of group-based CBT for chronic posttraumatic headache after mTBI showed a minor effect on quality of life, psychological distress, and overall experience of symptoms, and no effect on headache and pressure pain thresholds.[68]
- In children, most post-concussion symptoms resolve within a month after injury, the exception being children who have a history of previous head injury, learning difficulties, or family stressors, who are more likely to experience ongoing problems.[69] Ponsford and colleagues[70] demonstrated that an information booklet of strategies for dealing with posttraumatic symptoms resulted in fewer symptoms and less behavioral changes in children 3 months after injury.

Cognitive rehabilitation

- Studies of interventions to specifically improve cognition have indicated improvement in performance on selected neuropsychological (NP) test scores and cognitive functions following neurocognitive rehabilitation in patients with mild or mild-to-moderate TBI.[58,71,72] Neurocognitive rehabilitation uses cognitive tasks to improve cognitive processes, or it may involve developing compensatory strategies to address difficulties with aspects of cognition, such as attention, memory, and executive functioning.[9] Empirical support varies for neurocognitive rehabilitation of different cognitive processes. Neurocognitive rehabilitation of attention processes, which can affect memory, executive functioning, and other cognitive processes, has received the most empirical support with mTBI[58,71,73] and all severity levels of TBI.[74]

- A small RCT in mild to-moderate TBI of an 11-week program of combined neurocognitive rehabilitation and CBT improved divided auditory attention and levels of anxiety and depression in subjects who were symptomatic for 5 years.[75]
- Another recent trial compared supported employment along with a 12-week psychoeducation and compensatory cognitive training program to supported employment alone among veterans with mild to moderate TBI. The intervention group showed symptom reduction (Cohen d = 0.97) and improvement in prospective memory functioning (Cohen d = 0.72). Small-to-medium effect sizes were also found for posttraumatic stress disorder symptoms, depressive symptom severity, and attaining competitive work (Cohen d = 0.35–0.49).[76]

Physical therapy Symptoms after head injury are not specific to the brain.

- Concomitant injury to the cervical spine resembling whiplash may occur as a result of the acceleration-deceleration forces sustained in concussive trauma.[77]
- The upper cervical spine is particularly vulnerable to trauma because it is the most mobile part of the vertebral column with a complex proprioceptive system that has connections to the vestibular and visual systems.[78]
- Leslie and Craton[79] hypothesize that concussion is a syndrome that does not require brain involvement in all cases and that concussion-like symptoms can emanate from the cervical spine. In support of this, cervical spine injury has been associated with prolonged symptoms of headache, dizziness, blurred vision, and vertigo[80,81] as well as cognitive complaints, such as poor concentration and memory deficits.[82] Symptoms of headache, dizziness, poor concentration and memory, and vertigo may therefore result from either a brain injury, an injury to the cervical spine, or an injury to both.
- It is important for the clinician to establish as much as possible the mechanism of injury and perform a careful physical examination of the neck in all patients with PCS. If a cervical source is suspected to contribute to ongoing symptoms, it is recommended that therapy be instituted to treat abnormal neck position and movement sense as well as cervicogenic oculomotor disturbance, postural stability, and cervicogenic dizziness.[78] This recommendation is supported by 2 recent studies in SRC.
  - In a case series of elite athletes with persistent symptoms of dizziness, neck pain, and headaches after SRC, Schneider and colleagues[83] showed that a course of combined cervical spine manual therapy, neuromotor retraining, sensorimotor retraining, and vestibular physiotherapy produced functional and symptomatic improvements in all participants.
  - The same research group then performed an RCT of individuals with persistent symptoms of dizziness, neck pain, and headaches following SRC and found that participants undergoing the same active treatments were far more likely to be medically cleared to return to sport within 8 weeks of initiating treatment than the control group (risk ratio 10.3; 95% confidence interval 1.51–69.6).[83] Thus, active cervical and vestibular physical therapy can improve symptoms in patients suffering from prolonged symptoms after SRC and speed their return to sport.

Vestibular therapy Vestibular dysfunction is very common after concussion.

- The vestibular system is responsible for integrating information from head movements and limb position to maintain visual and balance control. It is a complex network that includes the inner ear, brainstem, cerebellum, cerebral cortex, ocular system, and postural muscles.[84]
- There are 2 basic divisions: the vestibulo-ocular system, which maintains visual stability during head movements, and the vestibulospinal system, which is responsible for postural control.[84]
- Injury or disease of the vestibulo-ocular system commonly manifests as symptoms of dizziness and visual instability. Conversely, vestibulospinal system dysfunction interferes with balance.[85] Vestibular dysfunction is commonly associated with TBI[86] and has been reported to delay recovery from concussion.[87,88] Dizziness, which may represent an underlying impairment of the vestibular and/or ocular motor systems, is reported by 50% of concussed athletes[89] and is associated with a 6.4 times greater risk, relative to any other on-field symptom, for predicting protracted recovery (ie, >21 days).[90]
- In a recent retrospective study of children and adolescents referred to a multidisciplinary pediatric concussion program, 28.6% with acute SRC and 62.5% of those with PCS met the clinical criteria for vestibulo-ocular dysfunction, which was a significant risk factor for the subsequent development of PCS in pediatric patients acutely after SRC.[91]
- Vestibular suppressants may delay recovery and have been supplanted by vestibular rehabilitation in the management of post-traumatic vertigo.[92] Vestibular rehabilitation can reduce dizziness and improve gait and balance function after concussion in both children and adults and should be considered in the management of individuals who have vestibular dysfunction after concussion.[86]
- As noted above, an RCT of individuals with persistent symptoms following SRC, including dizziness, found that participants were more likely to be medically cleared to return to sport within 8 weeks of initiating treatment with combined vestibular and cervical physiotherapy.[83]

Ocular therapy Ocular motor dysfunction is very common after concussion.

- The cognitive control of eye movements requires pathways involving fronto–parietal circuits and subcortical nuclei, many of which are particularly vulnerable to concussion.[93]
- Common neuro-ophthalmic findings in concussion include abnormalities in saccades (the eye's ability to quickly and accurately shift from one target to another); antisaccades (voluntary control over saccade direction to make the response in the opposite direction); smooth pursuits (slower tracking movements to keep a moving stimulus centered on the fovea); vergence (turning motion of the eyeballs toward or away from each other to maintain single binocular vision); accommodation (the ability of the eye to adjust its focal length and maintain focus); the vestibular–ocular reflex (reflex eye movement that stabilizes images on the retina during head movement), and photosensitivity.[93]
- Nearly 30% of concussed athletes report visual problems during the first week after injury,[89] and a recent study showed that 69% of adolescents after concussion (from within 1 month to more than 3 months from injury) had one or more of the following vision diagnoses: accommodative disorders (51%), convergence insufficiency (49%), or saccadic dysfunction (29%).[94]

- Symptoms of oculomotor dysfunction include double vision, blurry vision, headache, or difficulty with reading or other visual work, such as the use of a tablet, smartphone, or computer monitor in the school setting.[94]
- RCTs in the general population without concussion have demonstrated the effectiveness of vergence/accommodative therapy for the treatment of convergence insufficiency and accommodative insufficiency.[95–97]
- With respect to the treatment of visual symptoms after concussion in adults, a preliminary placebo controlled trial showed that oculomotor training (OMT) therapy improved rhythmicity, accuracy, and sequencing of saccades following mTBI (as a result of oculomotor learning).[98] There was also a significant reduction in near vision-related symptoms, increased visual attention, and improved reading ability in the OMT but not the placebo arm of the study.

Aerobic exercise therapy Autonomic dysfunction is present after concussion.[13]

- The Zurich Guidelines advise that when asymptomatic at rest, concussed patients should progress stepwise from light aerobic activity such as walking or stationary cycling up to sport or work-specific activities.[8] Athletes should not return-to-sport (RTS) until they can participate to the full extent of their sport without symptoms.
- Exercise intolerance may be a physiological sign or biomarker of ongoing concussion and the return of normal exercise tolerance may serve as a physiological biomarker to establish physiological recovery from concussion and readiness to RTS.[99]
- Leddy and colleagues[53] have applied this principle to those with persistent symptoms. Their preliminary studies show that individualized subthreshold aerobic exercise treatment improved symptoms in PCS subjects in association with improved fitness and autonomic function (ie, better heart rate [HR] and blood pressure [BP] control) during exercise and, when compared with a period of no intervention, safely sped recovery and restored function (ie, sport and work).[53,55]
- A similar rehabilitation program has been effective for children with PCS.[100]
- Recent fMRI imaging data suggest that some concussion symptoms may be related to abnormal local CBF regulation that is amenable to individualized aerobic exercise treatment. In a small placebo-controlled trial of PCS patients, subthreshold aerobic exercise treatment restored exercise tolerance to normal and brain fMRI activation patterns to controls levels, whereas subjects who received a placebo intervention did not.[101] The mechanisms for concussion-related exercise intolerance and for the effect of subthreshold exercise treatment in patients with concussion and PCS require further study.

The Buffalo Concussion Treadmill Test

- The Buffalo Concussion Treadmill Test (BCTT) is a standardized exercise test that is based on the Balke cardiac protocol. It imparts a gradual increase in workload and is the only functional test thus far shown to safely[53] and reliably[54] reveal physiological dysfunction in concussion, assist in the differential diagnosis of concussion from other diagnoses (eg, cervical injury, depression, migraines),[19] and quantify the clinical severity and exercise capacity of concussed patients.[53]
- The starting speed is 3.2 to 3.6 mph (depending on patient's age and height) at 0% incline. The incline is increased by 1% at minute 2 and by 1% each minute thereafter while maintaining the same speed until the subject cannot continue.
- The BCTT is stopped at the subjective report of significant symptom exacerbation (defined as ≥ 3 point increase over the pretreadmill test resting overall

symptom score on a 1- to 10-point visual analog scale, where a point is given for each increase in a symptom or the appearance of a new symptom) or at exhaustion (rating of perceived exertion [RPE] $\geq$17).[18] The HR recorded at the threshold of symptom exacerbation forms the basis for the individualized exercise prescription (see later discussion).

- Testing requires some experience because neurologic symptoms have been reported by healthy individuals following intense exercise,[102] and cervical symptoms and migraine headaches occasionally become exacerbated during the final stages of the test. The onset of symptom exacerbation in patients with physiological concussion occurs, however, much earlier in the test protocol and well short of predicted maximum exercise capacity.[18]
- The contraindications to performing the BCTT are those that would typically contraindicate the performance of a cardiac stress test and are presented in **Table 1**. Using the BCTT, the author has shown that it is safe for adult PCS patients to exercise up to 74% of maximum predicted capacity,[36] which provides an evidence base for stage 2 (light aerobic exercise) of the Zurich Conference Guidelines' graduated RTP protocol.[8]
- If a submaximal symptom exacerbation threshold is identified, patients are given a prescription to perform aerobic exercise (on a stationary cycle at first, to avoid the vestibular aspects of running) for 20 minutes per day at an intensity of 80% (90% in elite athletes) of the threshold HR achieved on the BCTT (this becomes the target HR) once per day for 5 to 6 days per week using an HR monitor.
- Patients are advised to terminate exercise at the first sign of symptom exacerbation or after 20 minutes, whichever comes first.
- Athletes should use an HR monitor so that they do not exceed the target HR exercise "dose."

Table 1
Absolute and relative contraindications to the Buffalo Concussion Treadmill Test

Absolute Contraindications	
History	Unwilling to exercise
	Increased risk for cardiopulmonary disease as defined by the American College of Sports Medicine[a]
Physical examination	Focal neurologic deficit
	Significant balance deficit, visual deficit, or orthopedic injury that would represent a significant risk for walking/running on a treadmill
Relative contraindications	
History	β-Blocker use
	Major depression (may not comply with directions or prescription)
	Does not understand English
Physical examination	Minor balance deficit, visual deficit, or orthopedic injury that increases risk for walking/running on a treadmill
	Resting systolic BP >140 mm Hg or diastolic BP >90 mm Hg
	Obesity: body mass index $\geq$30 kg/m^2

[a] Individuals with known cardiovascular, pulmonary, or metabolic disease; signs and symptoms suggestive of cardiovascular or pulmonary disease; or individuals $\geq$ age 45 who have more than one risk factor to include: (1) family history of myocardial infarction, coronary revascularization, or sudden death before 55 years of age; (2) cigarette smoking; (3) hypertension; (4) hypercholesterolemia; (5) impaired fasting glucose; or (6) obesity (body mass index $\geq$30 kg/m^2).

From Leddy JJ, Willer B. Use of graded exercise testing in concussion and return-to-activity management. Curr Sports Med Rep 2013;12(6):372; with permission.

- The BCTT can be repeated every 2 to 3 weeks to establish a new target HR until symptoms are no longer exacerbated during exercise. A more cost-effective approach, however, is simply to establish the subthreshold HR on the initial test and increase the exercise target HR by 5 to 10 bpm every 2 weeks (via phone call or e-mail), provided the patient is responding favorably.[18]
- More fit patients and athletes generally respond faster[53] and can increase their HR by 10 bpm every 1 to 2 weeks, whereas nonathletes typically respond better to 5 bpm increments every 2 weeks. Rate of exercise intensity progression varies, and some patients may have to stay at a particular HR for more than 2 weeks.
- Physiological resolution of concussion is defined as the ability to exercise to voluntary exhaustion at 85% to 90% of age-predicted maximum HR for 20 minutes without exacerbation of symptoms for several days in a row.[53] Patients can then begin the Zurich RTP program.
- Exercise testing should only be considered for patients without orthopedic or vestibular problems that increase the risk of falling and only in those patients who are at low risk for cardiac disease.[18] In those patients who have a different cause of persistent symptoms (eg, cervical or vestibulo-ocular disorders), or a combination of disorders (patients with physiological post-concussion disorder can also have a neck injury), the author has found that subthreshold exercise along with specific treatment of the concomitant disorder enhances recovery as well.[55]

SUMMARY

Traditionally, patients have been advised to restrict physical and cognitive activity after concussion until all symptoms resolve. Recent research, however, suggests that prolonged rest beyond the first couple of days after concussion might hinder rather than aid recovery and that a more active approach to concussion management should be considered. Humans do not respond well to removal from their social and physical environments. Sustained rest adversely affects the physiology of concussion and can lead to physical deconditioning and reactive depression. New research suggests that patients after concussion can safely engage in controlled physical activity below the symptom threshold and that controlled activity may even be beneficial to recovery. Practitioners should always take a careful history and perform a physical examination in patients with concussion and in those with delayed recovery to try to identify one or more potentially treatable post-concussion disorders. Several active treatments (eg, subthreshold aerobic exercise, cervical, vestibular, cognitive behavioral, and/or vision therapy) may improve recovery from concussion if they are implemented at the right time. The principle of exercise tolerance can be used to help with the differential diagnosis of PCS, and return of normal exercise tolerance can serve as a physiological biomarker of readiness to return to sport in athletes. Additional research should determine the appropriate timing, mode, duration, intensity, and frequency of exercise during the acute recovery phase of concussion before making specific exercise recommendations. Subsymptom threshold aerobic exercise improves activity tolerance and is an appropriate treatment option for patients with prolonged symptoms after concussion.

REFERENCES

1. Silverberg ND, Iverson GL. Is rest after concussion "the best medicine?": recommendations for activity resumption following concussion in athletes, civilians, and military service members. J Head Trauma Rehabil 2013;28(4):250–9.

2. Giza CC, Hovda DA. The neurometabolic cascade of concussion. J Athl Train 2001;36(3):228–35.
3. Longhi L, Saatman KE, Fujimoto S, et al. Temporal window of vulnerability to repetitive experimental concussive brain injury. Neurosurgery 2005;56(2):364–74 [discussion: 374].
4. Cantu RC. Second-impact syndrome. Clin Sports Med 1998;17(1):37–44.
5. McCrory PR, Berkovic SF. Second impact syndrome. Neurology 1998;50(3): 677–83.
6. Guskiewicz KM, McCrea M, Marshall SW, et al. Cumulative effects associated with recurrent concussion in collegiate football players: the NCAA concussion study. JAMA 2003;290(19):2549–55.
7. Majerske CW, Mihalik JP, Ren D, et al. Concussion in sports: postconcussive activity levels, symptoms, and neurocognitive performance. J Athl Train 2008; 43(3):265–74.
8. McCrory P, Meeuwisse W, Aubry M, et al. Consensus statement on concussion in sport–the 4th International Conference on Concussion in Sport held in Zurich, November 2012. Clin J Sport Med 2013;23(2):89–117.
9. Leddy JJ, Sandhu H, Sodhi V, et al. Rehabilitation of concussion and post-concussion syndrome. Sports Health 2012;4(2):147–54.
10. Thomas DG, Apps JN, Hoffmann RG, et al. Benefits of strict rest after acute concussion: a randomized controlled trial. Pediatrics 2015;135(2):213–23.
11. McKeag DB, Kutcher JS. Concussion consensus: raising the bar and filling in the gaps. Clin J Sport Med 2009;19(5):343–6.
12. Bazarian JJ. Diagnosing mild traumatic brain injury after a concussion. J Head Trauma Rehabil 2010;25(4):225–7.
13. Leddy JJ, Kozlowski K, Fung M, et al. Regulatory and autoregulatory physiological dysfunction as a primary characteristic of post concussion syndrome: implications for treatment. NeuroRehabilitation 2007;22(3):199–205.
14. Henry LC, Elbin RJ, Collins MW, et al. Examining recovery trajectories after sport-related concussion with a multimodal clinical assessment approach. Neurosurgery 2015;78(2):232–41.
15. Al Sayegh A, Sandford D, Carson AJ. Psychological approaches to treatment of postconcussion syndrome: a systematic review. J Neurol Neurosurg Psychiatry 2010;81(10):1128–34.
16. Dimberg EL, Burns TM. Management of common neurologic conditions in sports. Clin Sports Med 2005;24(3):637–62, ix.
17. Kutcher JS, Eckner JT. At-risk populations in sports-related concussion. Curr Sports Med Rep 2010;9(1):16–20.
18. Leddy JJ, Willer B. Use of graded exercise testing in concussion and return-to-activity management. Curr Sports Med Rep 2013;12(6):370–6.
19. Leddy JJ, Baker JG, Merchant A, et al. Brain or strain? Symptoms alone do not distinguish physiologic concussion from cervical/vestibular injury. Clin J Sport Med 2015;25(3):237–42.
20. Binder LM, Rohling ML, Larrabee GJ. A review of mild head trauma. Part I: meta-analytic review of neuropsychological studies. J Clin Exp Neuropsychol 1997; 19(3):421–31.
21. Rimel RW, Giordani B, Barth JT, et al. Disability caused by minor head injury. Neurosurgery 1981;9(3):221–8.
22. McCauley SR, Boake C, Levin HS, et al. Postconcussional disorder following mild to moderate traumatic brain injury: anxiety, depression, and social support as risk factors and comorbidities. J Clin Exp Neuropsychol 2001;23(6):792–808.

23. Iverson GL, Gaetz M, Lovell MR, et al. Cumulative effects of concussion in amateur athletes. Brain Inj 2004;18(5):433–43.
24. McCrory P, Johnston K, Meeuwisse W, et al. Summary and agreement statement of the 2nd International Conference on Concussion in Sport, Prague 2004. Clin J Sport Med 2005;15(2):48–55.
25. De Kruijk JR, Twijnstra A, Meerhoff S, et al. Management of mild traumatic brain injury: lack of consensus in Europe. Brain Inj 2001;15(2):117–23.
26. Chen JK, Johnston KM, Frey S, et al. Functional abnormalities in symptomatic concussed athletes: an fMRI study. Neuroimage 2004;22(1):68–82.
27. Jantzen KJ. Functional magnetic resonance imaging of mild traumatic brain injury. J Head Trauma Rehabil 2010;25(4):256–66.
28. Brown NJ, Mannix RC, O'Brien MJ, et al. Effect of cognitive activity level on duration of post-concussion symptoms. Pediatrics 2014;133(2):e299–304.
29. Lovell MR, Iverson GL, Collins MW, et al. Measurement of symptoms following sports-related concussion: reliability and normative data for the post-concussion scale. Appl Neuropsychol 2006;13(3):166–74.
30. de Kruijk JR, Leffers P, Meerhoff S, et al. Effectiveness of bed rest after mild traumatic brain injury: a randomised trial of no versus six days of bed rest. J Neurol Neurosurg Psychiatry 2002;73(2):167–72.
31. Clausen M, Pendergast DR, Willer B, et al. Cerebral blood flow during treadmill exercise is a marker of physiological postconcussion syndrome in female athletes. J Head Trauma Rehabil 2015. [Epub ahead of print].
32. Maugans TA, Farley C, Altaye M, et al. Pediatric sports-related concussion produces cerebral blood flow alterations. Pediatrics 2012;129(1):28–37.
33. Meier TB, Bellgowan PS, Singh R, et al. Recovery of cerebral blood flow following sports-related concussion. JAMA Neurol 2015;72(5):530–8.
34. Zhang R, Zuckerman JH, Pawelczyk JA, et al. Effects of head-down-tilt bed rest on cerebral hemodynamics during orthostatic stress. J Appl Physiol (1985) 1997;83(6):2139–45.
35. Guiney H, Lucas SJ, Cotter JD, et al. Evidence cerebral blood-flow regulation mediates exercise-cognition links in healthy young adults. Neuropsychology 2014;29(1):1–9.
36. Kozlowski KF, Graham J, Leddy JJ, et al. Exercise intolerance in individuals with postconcussion syndrome. J Athl Train 2013;48(5):627–35.
37. Carson JD, Lawrence DW, Kraft SA, et al. Premature return to play and return to learn after a sport-related concussion: physician's chart review. Can Fam Physician 2014;60(6):e310, e312–5.
38. Satterthwaite TD, Shinohara RT, Wolf DH, et al. Impact of puberty on the evolution of cerebral perfusion during adolescence. Proc Natl Acad Sci U S A 2014; 111(23):8643–8.
39. Willer B, Leddy JJ. Management of concussion and post-concussion syndrome. Curr Treat Options Neurol 2006;8(5):415–26.
40. Buckley TA, Munkasy BA, Clouse BP. Acute cognitive and physical rest may not improve concussion recovery time. J Head Trauma Rehabil 2015. [Epub ahead of print].
41. Hou R, Moss-Morris R, Peveler R, et al. When a minor head injury results in enduring symptoms: a prospective investigation of risk factors for postconcussional syndrome after mild traumatic brain injury. J Neurol Neurosurg Psychiatry 2012;83(2):217–23.
42. McAllister TW, Arciniegas D. Evaluation and treatment of postconcussive symptoms. NeuroRehabilitation 2002;17(4):265–83.

43. Griesbach GS, Hovda DA, Molteni R, et al. Voluntary exercise following traumatic brain injury: brain-derived neurotrophic factor upregulation and recovery of function. Neuroscience 2004;125(1):129–39.
44. Griesbach GS, Tio DL, Nair S, et al. Temperature and heart rate responses to exercise following mild traumatic brain injury. J Neurotrauma 2013;30(4): 281–91.
45. Griesbach GS, Tio DL, Nair S, et al. Recovery of stress response coincides with responsiveness to voluntary exercise after traumatic brain injury. J Neurotrauma 2014;31(7):674–82.
46. Griesbach GS, Tio DL, Vincelli J, et al. Differential effects of voluntary and forced exercise on stress responses after traumatic brain injury. J Neurotrauma 2012; 29(7):1426–33.
47. Itoh T, Imano M, Nishida S, et al. Exercise inhibits neuronal apoptosis and improves cerebral function following rat traumatic brain injury. J Neural Transm 2011;118(9):1263–72.
48. Itoh T, Imano M, Nishida S, et al. Exercise increases neural stem cell proliferation surrounding the area of damage following rat traumatic brain injury. J Neural Transm 2011;118(2):193–202.
49. Jacotte-Simancas A, Costa-Miserachs D, Coll-Andreu M, et al. Effects of voluntary physical exercise, citicoline, and combined treatment on object recognition memory, neurogenesis, and neuroprotection after traumatic brain injury in rats. J Neurotrauma 2015;32(10):739–51.
50. Seo TB, Kim BK, Ko IG, et al. Effect of treadmill exercise on Purkinje cell loss and astrocytic reaction in the cerebellum after traumatic brain injury. Neurosci Lett 2010;481(3):178–82.
51. Hamilton MT, Hamilton DG, Zderic TW. Exercise physiology versus inactivity physiology: an essential concept for understanding lipoprotein lipase regulation. Exerc Sport Sci Rev 2004;32(4):161–6.
52. Berlin AA, Kop WJ, Deuster PA. Depressive mood symptoms and fatigue after exercise withdrawal: the potential role of decreased fitness. Psychosom Med 2006;68(2):224–30.
53. Leddy JJ, Kozlowski K, Donnelly JP, et al. A preliminary study of subsymptom threshold exercise training for refractory post-concussion syndrome. Clin J Sport Med 2010;20(1):21–7.
54. Leddy JJ, Baker JG, Kozlowski K, et al. Reliability of a graded exercise test for assessing recovery from concussion. Clin J Sport Med 2011;21(2):89–94.
55. Baker JG, Freitas MS, Leddy JJ, et al. Return to full functioning after graded exercise assessment and progressive exercise treatment of postconcussion syndrome. Rehabil Res Pract 2012;2012:705309.
56. Conder R, Conder AA. Neuropsychological and psychological rehabilitation interventions in refractory sport-related post-concussive syndrome. Brain Inj 2015;29(2):249–62.
57. Silver JM. Neuropsychiatry of persistent symptoms after concussion. Psychiatr Clin North Am 2014;37(1):91–102.
58. Helmick K, Members of Consensus Conference. Cognitive rehabilitation for military personnel with mild traumatic brain injury and chronic post-concussional disorder: results of April 2009 consensus conference. NeuroRehabilitation 2010;26(3):239–55.
59. Potter S, Brown RG. Cognitive behavioural therapy and persistent post-concussional symptoms: integrating conceptual issues and practical aspects in treatment. Neuropsychol Rehabil 2012;22(1):1–25.

60. Mittenberg W, Canyock EM, Condit D, et al. Treatment of post-concussion syndrome following mild head injury. J Clin Exp Neuropsychol 2001;23(6):829–36.

61. Ponsford J, Willmott C, Rothwell A, et al. Impact of early intervention on outcome following mild head injury in adults. J Neurol Neurosurg Psychiatry 2002;73(3): 330–2.

62. Mittenberg W, Tremont G, Zielinski RE, et al. Cognitive-behavioral prevention of postconcussion syndrome. Arch Clin Neuropsychol 1996;11(2):139–45.

63. Wade DT, King NS, Wenden FJ, et al. Routine follow up after head injury: a second randomised controlled trial. J Neurol Neurosurg Psychiatry 1998;65(2): 177–83.

64. Andersson EE, Emanuelson I, Bjorklund R, et al. Mild traumatic brain injuries: the impact of early intervention on late sequelae. A randomized controlled trial. Acta Neurochir (Wien) 2007;149:151–60.

65. Ghaffar O, McCullagh S, Ouchterlony D, et al. Randomized treatment trial in mild traumatic brain injury. J Psychosom Res 2006;61(2):153–60.

66. Silverberg ND, Hallam BJ, Rose A, et al. Cognitive-behavioral prevention of postconcussion syndrome in at-risk patients: a pilot randomized controlled trial. J Head Trauma Rehabil 2013;28(4):313–22.

67. Whittaker R, Kemp S, House A. Illness perceptions and outcome in mild head injury: a longitudinal study. J Neurol Neurosurg Psychiatry 2007;78(6):644–6.

68. Kjeldgaard D, Forchhammer HB, Teasdale TW, et al. Cognitive behavioural treatment for the chronic post-traumatic headache patient: a randomized controlled trial. J Headache Pain 2014;15:81.

69. Ponsford J, Willmott C, Rothwell A, et al. Cognitive and behavioral outcome following mild traumatic head injury in children. J Head Trauma Rehabil 1999; 14(4):360–72.

70. Ponsford J, Willmott C, Rothwell A, et al. Impact of early intervention on outcome after mild traumatic brain injury in children. Pediatrics 2001;108(6):1297–303.

71. Cicerone KD. Remediation of "working attention" in mild traumatic brain injury. Brain Inj 2002;16(3):185–95.

72. Ho MR, Bennett TL. Efficacy of neuropsychological rehabilitation for mild-moderate traumatic brain injury. Arch Clin Neuropsychol 1997;12(1):1–11.

73. Palmese CA, Raskin SA. The rehabilitation of attention in individuals with mild traumatic brain injury, using the APT-II programme. Brain Inj 2000;14(6):535–48.

74. Rohling ML, Faust ME, Beverly B, et al. Effectiveness of cognitive rehabilitation following acquired brain injury: a meta-analytic re-examination of Cicerone et al.'s (2000, 2005) systematic reviews. Neuropsychology 2009;23(1):20–39.

75. Tiersky LA, Anselmi V, Johnston MV, et al. A trial of neuropsychologic rehabilitation in mild-spectrum traumatic brain injury. Arch Phys Med Rehabil 2005;86(8): 1565–74.

76. Twamley EW, Jak AJ, Delis DC, et al. Cognitive Symptom Management And Rehabilitation Therapy (CogSMART) for veterans with traumatic brain injury: pilot randomized controlled trial. J Rehabil Res Dev 2014;51(1):59–70.

77. Barth JT, Freeman JR, Broshek DK, et al. Acceleration-deceleration sport-related concussion: the gravity of it all. J Athl Train 2001;36(3):253–6.

78. Kristjansson E, Treleaven J. Sensorimotor function and dizziness in neck pain: implications for assessment and management. J Orthop Sports Phys Ther 2009;39(5):364–77.

79. Leslie O, Craton N. Concussion: purely a brain injury? Clin J Sport Med 2013; 23(5):331–2.

80. Endo K, Ichimaru K, Komagata M, et al. Cervical vertigo and dizziness after whiplash injury. Eur Spine J 2006;15(6):886–90.

81. Treleaven J. Dizziness, unsteadiness, visual disturbances, and postural control: implications for the transition to chronic symptoms after a whiplash trauma. Spine (Phila Pa 1976) 2011;36(25 Suppl):S211–7.

82. Sturzenegger M, Radanov BP, Winter P, et al. MRI-based brain volumetry in chronic whiplash patients: no evidence for traumatic brain injury. Acta Neurol Scand 2008;117(1):49–54.

83. Schneider KJ, Iverson GL, Emery CA, et al. The effects of rest and treatment following sport-related concussion: a systematic review of the literature. Br J Sports Med 2013;47(5):304–7.

84. Cullen KE. The vestibular system: multimodal integration and encoding of self-motion for motor control. Trends Neurosci 2012;35(3):185–96.

85. Khan S, Chang R. Anatomy of the vestibular system: a review. NeuroRehabilitation 2013;32(3):437–43.

86. Alsalaheen BA, Mucha A, Morris LO, et al. Vestibular rehabilitation for dizziness and balance disorders after concussion. J Neurol Phys Ther 2010;34(2):87–93.

87. Hoffer ME, Gottshall KR, Moore R, et al. Characterizing and treating dizziness after mild head trauma. Otol Neurotol 2004;25(2):135–8.

88. Naguib MB, Madian Y, Refaat M, et al. Characterisation and objective monitoring of balance disorders following head trauma, using videonystagmography. J Laryngol Otol 2012;126(1):26–33.

89. Kontos AP, Elbin RJ, Schatz P, et al. A revised factor structure for the post-concussion symptom scale: baseline and postconcussion factors. Am J Sports Med 2012;40(10):2375–84.

90. Lau BC, Kontos AP, Collins MW, et al. Which on-field signs/symptoms predict protracted recovery from sport-related concussion among high school football players? Am J Sports Med 2011;39(11):2311–8.

91. Ellis MJ, Cordingley D, Vis S, et al. Vestibulo-ocular dysfunction in pediatric sports-related concussion. J Neurosurg Pediatr 2015;16(3):248–55.

92. Friedman JM. Post-traumatic vertigo. Med Health R I 2004;87(10):296–300.

93. Ventura RE, Jancuska JM, Balcer LJ, et al. Diagnostic tests for concussion: is vision part of the puzzle? J Neuroophthalmol 2015;35(1):73–81.

94. Master CL, Scheiman M, Gallaway M, et al. Vision diagnoses are common after concussion in adolescents. Clin Pediatr (Phila) 2015;1–8.

95. Scheiman M. Treatment of symptomatic convergence insufficiency in children with a home-based computer orthoptic exercise program. J AAPOS 2011; 15(2):123–4.

96. Scheiman M, Cotter S, Kulp MT, et al. Treatment of accommodative dysfunction in children: results from a randomized clinical trial. Optom Vis Sci 2011;88(11): 1343–52.

97. Scheiman M, Cotter S, Rouse M, et al. Randomised clinical trial of the effectiveness of base-in prism reading glasses versus placebo reading glasses for symptomatic convergence insufficiency in children. Br J Ophthalmol 2005; 89(10):1318–23.

98. Thiagarajan P, Ciuffreda KJ. Effect of oculomotor rehabilitation on vergence responsivity in mild traumatic brain injury. J Rehabil Res Dev 2013;50(9):1223–40.

99. Darling SR, Leddy JJ, Baker JG, et al. Evaluation of the Zurich guidelines and exercise testing for return to play in adolescents following concussion. Clin J Sport Med 2014;24(2):128–33.

100. Gagnon I, Galli C, Friedman D, et al. Active rehabilitation for children who are slow to recover following sport-related concussion. Brain Inj 2009;23(12): 956–64.
101. Leddy JJ, Cox JL, Baker JG, et al. Exercise treatment for postconcussion syndrome: a pilot study of changes in functional magnetic resonance imaging activation, physiology, and symptoms. J Head Trauma Rehabil 2013;28(4):241–9.
102. Alla S, Sullivan SJ, McCrory P, et al. Does exercise evoke neurological symptoms in healthy subjects? J Sci Med Sport 2010;13(1):24–6.

Managing Patients with Prolonged Recovery Following Concussion

Mary Miller Phillips, MD, Cara Camiolo Reddy, MD, MMM*

KEYWORDS

- Concussion • Postconcussion syndrome • Pharmacologic interventions
- Non-pharmacologic management

KEY POINTS

- Persistent symptoms following concussion can be challenging for clinicians, given variable presentations among patients.
- A thorough history and physical examination are key to developing a treatment approach.
- Pharmacologic treatments can be considered when symptoms are negatively affecting quality of life.

INTRODUCTION

Concussion awareness, particularly in sports, has significantly increased over the past decade, and the body of literature regarding diagnostic criteria, evaluation, management, risk factors, prognosis, and long-term effects has grown exponentially. Recommendations for acute concussion management emphasize physical and cognitive rest balanced with supervised graded exertion until symptoms resolve before return to play.[1–3] Although this approach is effective in most patients with concussion, it is estimated that the incidence of postconcussion syndrome (PCS) can range from 1.4% to 29.3% among different populations evaluated using inconsistent diagnostic criteria.[4–7]

Persistent symptoms following concussion can be debilitating for patients and challenging for clinicians, given the limited data available on the management of prolonged recovery from concussion. PCS refers to the collection of symptoms across several clinical domains that occur after concussion. Symptoms may include headache, nausea, dizziness, impaired balance, blurred vision, confusion, memory impairment, mental "fogginess," and fatigue, in varying combinations.[8–13] Although evidence-based approaches are emerging, issues related to the diagnostic criteria continue

Brain Injury Program, Department of Physical Medicine and Rehabilitation, UPMC Rehabilitation Institute, University of Pittsburgh Medical Center, 1400 Locust Street, D-G103, Pittsburgh, PA 15219, USA
* Corresponding author.
E-mail address: camice@upmc.edu

Phys Med Rehabil Clin N Am 27 (2016) 455–474
http://dx.doi.org/10.1016/j.pmr.2015.12.005
1047-9651/16/$ – see front matter

to complicate the literature and clinical identification. The *Diagnostic and Statistical Manual of Mental Disorders, Fifth Edition*, and *International Classification of Diseases, 10th Revision*, both provide criteria for the diagnosis of PCS; however, Rose and colleagues[14] were able to demonstrate ongoing variability among practitioners by using an electronic survey. Another challenge to developing strict diagnostic criteria is that symptoms seen following PCS also have been reported in a variety of other diagnoses, such as uninjured controls, patients with general trauma, personal injury claimants, soldiers with combat stress, patients suffering from depression/anxiety, and patients with chronic pain.[15–19]

PATHOPHYSIOLOGY

Concussion is a complex pathophysiological process affecting the brain, induced by traumatic biomechanical forces.[1–3] Following impact, the brain experiences a complex cascade of ionic, metabolic, and physiologic events, well described by Giza and Hovda.[20] Indiscriminate release of excitatory amino acids, coupled with a massive efflux of potassium, induces a brief period of hyperglycolysis. This is in response to ATP-powered sodium-potassium pumps operating at maximum capacity in attempts to restore neuronal membrane potential. The hypermetabolic state occurs in the setting of diminished cerebral blood flow causing a cellular "energy crisis," as the supply of glucose cannot meet the demand. What follows is a period of depressed metabolism secondary to persistent calcium influx causing mitochondrial dysfunction and impaired oxidative metabolism. ATP consumption and production become unbalanced, thus worsening the energy crisis. In the later stages of the cascade, the balance between glucose metabolism and cerebral blood flow is restored, but delayed cell death, chronic alterations in neurotransmission, and axonal disconnection occur.[20] The metabolic derangement and the postconcussion "energy crisis" are considered chiefly responsible for the compromised synaptic plasticity and subsequent cognitive deficits.[21] Clinical signs and symptoms of concussion, such as impaired coordination, attention, memory, and cognition are manifestations of underlying neuronal dysfunction, likely due to the processes described.[20]

Using animal models, Rathbone and colleagues[22] described the potential role systemic inflammation may have regarding symptoms of PCS. These models have demonstrated activation of immune and nonimmune cells and increases in inflammatory mediators (ie, cytokines) following brain injury. Microglia, which become activated after injury, appear to be an important component of the long-term inflammatory response. Once activated, they release immune factors, such as reactive oxygen species, prostaglandins, and excitotoxins.[22–24] The role of inflammation in headache, irritability, anxiety and depression, personality changes, apathy, sleep disturbance, fatigue, and reduced tolerance to stress has been described via literature review in animal and human subjects with no history of head injury.[22] These symptoms are commonly reported in PCS and it may be postulated that PCS following concussion represents a "persistent, low-grade, chronically smoldering neuroinflammatory response."[22,24]

RISK FACTORS FOR PROLONGED RECOVERY

It has been stated that recovery from concussion occurs within a relatively short time frame, with more than 90% of injured athletes returning to play within 7 to 14 days after injury.[4,25] However, recent work by Henry and colleagues[26] evaluated 66 subjects (64% male, ages 14–23 years) and found that although the greatest rate of symptom improvement occurred in the first 2 weeks after injury, recovery time across all symptoms, neurocognitive and vestibular-ocular outcomes happened by 21 to 28 days after injury.

Literature regarding specific risk factors for the development of PCS is conflicting. This is likely due to the varied nature of postconcussive symptoms and the subjectivity of symptom reporting. Variables, such as genetics, mental health history, life stressors, medical problems, chronic pain, depression, personality factors, and other psychosocial and environmental factors, may play an influential role.[16,19,27–29] The presence of premorbid psychiatric illnesses, such as anxiety, depression, and compulsive, histrionic, and narcissistic personality disorders or those with a family history of mood disorder have been found to have higher incidence of PCS.[30] Negative perceptions of concussion and "all or nothing" personality types were found to be correlated with prolonged recoveries.[31] Patients with histories of premorbid learning disorders or attention deficits may experience exacerbation of baseline symptoms after concussion.[32] Additionally, practitioners may experience difficulty interpreting results of neuropsychological testing if no baseline testing was performed, due to questions about which abnormalities are new or were preexisting.[33] Signs and symptoms immediately following impact and their association with recovery patterns have been described by several studies.[9,34–36] Most recently, Lau and colleagues[36] followed 107 high school football players from time of impact to return to play so as to determine which on-field signs and symptoms were predictive of a protracted (>21 days) versus rapid (<7 days) recovery. On-field signs and symptoms included confusion, loss of consciousness, posttraumatic amnesia, retrograde amnesia, imbalance, dizziness, visual problems, personality changes, fatigue, sensitivity to light/noise, numbness, and vomiting. Dizziness was found to have the strongest correlation with a protracted recovery, whereas the remaining signs and symptoms were not predictive of prolonged recoveries. In the days after concussion, fogginess, memory impairment, anxiety, and noise sensitivity also have been identified as risk factors for persistent postconcussion symptoms.[9,36,37]

There are conflicting data regarding the association between female gender and increased risk of developing PCS. Dick and colleagues[38] and McCauley and colleagues[39] identified female gender as a risk factor for development of PCS compared with male counterparts. Farace and colleagues[40] also found that women had poorer outcomes across 85% of variables used in a meta-analysis of 20 clinical outcomes. In another study of female and male soccer players, female athletes reported more symptoms and neurocognitive impairment compared with their male counterparts.[41] However, outcome studies suggest that differences reported between genders may be limited, as women may be more inclined to report symptoms than men.[38]

There may be a relationship between the number of previously sustained concussions and the development of PCS. Evidence exists that athletes who have sustained previous concussions experience prolonged recovery patterns in comparison with their counterparts who have not had previous concussions.[42–44] Additionally, 2 studies reported findings of poor executive function and information processing speed in high school and college athletes with 2 or more previous concussions.[45,46] However, alternative studies have shown no relationship,[47,48] and this continues to be an area of uncertainty.

Finally, genetic influences on outcomes following concussion have been studied. The *APOE* gene (located on chromosome 9 at position q13.2) produces apolipoprotein E (ApoE), which assists with lipid transport in the brain, maintains neural integrity, and assists with recovery after brain injury.[49,50] After injury, production of ApoE increases with ApoE-epsilon 4 (allele of ApoE) inhibiting neurite outgrowth. ApoE-epsilon 4 has been identified as a risk factor for Alzheimer disease[51] and is associated with worse functional and cognitive outcomes after severe traumatic brain injury.[52,53] Based on current research, the presence of ApoE-epsilon 4 does not appear to prognosticate a worse outcome following concussion[54–56]; however, preliminary research is suggesting that individuals with the *APOE* promoter G-219T-TT genotype may be predisposed to concussion.[57] Currently, no genetic screening test is available for routine use in the clinical setting.

EFFECTS OF MULTIPLE CONCUSSIONS

In general, the prognosis is good for full recovery after sustaining a single concussion and many individuals will have spontaneous symptom resolution without further sequelae; however, evidence is suggesting that there may be long-term consequences in individuals who sustain multiple concussions. Athletes who have sustained multiple concussions may be at risk for sustaining additional concussions during the recovery period and the second injury may be the result of a relatively mild impact.[42] The most concerning, albeit rare, consequence of repeated head injury during the acute phase is the second impact syndrome (SIS). Initially described in 1973, SIS occurs when a second concussive impact is sustained before symptoms of the initial impact have fully resolved, causing rapid and catastrophic brain swelling that is severely disabling and typically fatal.[58]

Chronic effects of multiple concussions in younger individuals continue to be a subject of debate. In studies of high school/collegiate athletes with histories of multiple concussions, no neuropsychological deficits were demonstrated 6 months after concussion[59,60]; however, other studies have shown lower baseline testing; neuropsychological deficits in memory, planning, and visuo-perceptual tasks; and increased vulnerability to repeated concussions in athletes who have sustained multiple concussions.[61–63]

Studies performed using older, former athletes who have sustained multiple concussions describe relationships between number of concussions sustained and findings of impaired neurocognitive performance in episodic memory and response inhibition, neuroelectrophysiological alterations, higher than average rates of depression, and increasing risk of mild cognitive impairment (a condition that converts to Alzheimer disease at a rate of 10%–20% annually).[64–68]

Differences seen in younger versus older athletes who have sustained multiple concussions may be explained by the concept of "physiologic reserve."[69] Through recruitment of brain networks and/or alternative cognitive strategies, the brain is able to compensate for damage. Throughout a person's life, cognitive reserve is reduced due to damage from environmental, developmental, and genetic sources. This combined with accumulating brain damaging experiences and waning health as a result of aging leads to a decline in cognitive function. Younger athletes are likely able to rely on their cognitive reserve after multiple concussions, but this may not be the case over time.[69]

The long-term effects of repetitive subconcussive hits are less clear, as they are usually asymptomatic. Although conventional imaging studies (computed tomography, MRI) are negative for most concussions, in cases in which athletes sustain multiple hits to the head (ie, boxers), the presence of age-inappropriate volume loss, cavum septum pellucidum, and subcortical and periventricular white matter disease has been demonstrated[70,71] compared with controls. Cavum septum pellucidum has been speculated to be a marker of chronic brain trauma.[72]

There is no consensus regarding the decision of when to forgo high-contact sports/activities when multiple concussions have been sustained. It has been suggested that removal should be considered when the time between concussions is decreasing, symptoms are becoming more severe and prolonged with each subsequent injury, or when concussions are occurring with less and less force.[73]

EVALUATION

The evaluation of a patient with suspected PCS should always start with a thorough history. Components that should be assessed include mood and affect, structure and quality of thought, sleep, somatic symptoms (headache profile, vision, dizziness, balance, nausea/emesis), musculoskeletal pain (particularly cervical/trapezius pain associated with headaches), prescribed medication history (before and after injury), premorbid risk factors (particularly anxiety/depression, migraines, history of concussions, learning disabilities), family history of psychiatric/neurologic illness, substance abuse history, and history of self-injurious behavior or ideation.[74] It has also been recommended that the use of standardized symptom assessment scales be used.[75] Differential diagnoses should remain broad, as signs and symptoms of PCS can be seen with a variety of other diagnoses.

Physical examination should consist of a thorough neurologic examination of cognition, cranial nerve function, strength, sensation, reflexes, cerebellar function, and gait and balance. Cerebellar examination should include evaluations for appendicular ataxia, truncal ataxia, and eye movement abnormalities. Tests for appendicular ataxia include finger-nose-finger test, heel shin test, and rapid alternating movements. The examiner is looking for signs of dysrhythmia, dysmetria, or dysdiadochokinesia. The Romberg test and tandem gait evaluate for truncal ataxia, with loss of balance (usually toward the side of the lesion) considered positive. Finally, abnormalities of eye movements can be observed, including ocular dysmetria (saccades overshoot or undershoot their targets), nystagmus, and impairment of vestibule-ocular reflex (VOR) suppression. VOR testing consists of 2 parts: patient fixates on a static object while performing rapid horizontal/vertical head movements followed by fixation on a static object while rotating entire trunk. The patient should be able to maintain gaze on static object during dynamic movement without nystagmus. Examination of the cervical spine and neck musculature is indicated in complaints of neck pain and headaches, and whiplash syndrome should be considered.

Computed tomography is the imaging modality of choice in the acute care setting following possible concussive injury, and is abnormal in fewer than 10% of cases with 0.1% to 1% requiring surgical intervention.[76,77] Conventional MRI is often considered when symptoms are prolonged; however, the utility of MRI in concussion is debated. A normal MRI does not exclude concussion, as it is not sensitive enough to identify structural injury to axons consistently or detect ongoing metabolic abnormalities. Imaging modalities such as functional MRI, single-photon emission computed tomography, magnetic resonance spectroscopy, or magnetoencephalogram may be more appropriate for concussion, as they provide a better understanding of brain function rather than structure alone; however, they are not routinely used in clinical evaluation currently and their utility in identifying appropriate clinical interventions remains to be investigated.[78]

Finally, there is evidence that neuropsychological testing is useful in the evaluation of concussion, particularly for acute management decisions on the sideline and tracking recovery in the acute phase.[1,2,79] Although questions remain regarding which battery of tests to administer, in what form and at what time points, neuropsychological testing can be considered in the evaluation of the patient with persistent symptoms, particularly those with cognitive complaints.

GENERAL TREATMENT PRINCIPLES

As symptom presentations vary, treatment approaches should be tailored to the individual. Patient education and reassurance should be a primary intervention. Miller and Mittenberg[80] found that a single psychoeducational session is a key factor in preventing or shortening PCS. In the acute phase, a reasonable amount of cognitive and physical rest is recommended; however, it has been demonstrated that prolonged rest can be detrimental to recovery and should not be extended past the first few weeks following injury.[81,82] As patients begin their gradual return to activity, academic and work accommodations may be needed.

Meehan[83] described conditions in which pharmacologic intervention can be considered: when symptoms last longer than expected recovery time, quality of life is affected, and the clinician is knowledgeable in the management of brain injury. On initiation of medication management, physicians and patients need to set clear treatment goals, and close follow-up should be arranged. Polypharmacy should be avoided and medications should be started at low doses, given an appropriate amount of time to assess effectiveness and monitor for side effects with slow upward titration. If possible, medications that target more than one symptom and have favorable side-effect profiles should be used.

In the following sections, symptoms are divided into 4 classes for simplicity: sleep, somatic (posttraumatic headaches, vestibular-vision dysfunction), mood, and cognitive. However, it should be recognized that there can be considerable overlap in symptom presentations that change over time, as explored by Kontos and colleagues[84] using factor analysis of symptom reporting on the Post Concussion Symptom Scale before and after injury (up to 7 days).

Sleep

Sleep disturbance is a common complaint following all severities of traumatic brain injuries (TBIs). Up to 70% of patients with TBI report sleep-wake cycle disruption (difficulty falling asleep or staying asleep), 33% report fatigue, and 10% report insomnia/excessive daytime sleepiness.[85,86] Many factors can contribute to sleep disturbance, including the injury itself, medication side effects, pain, preexisting sleep disorders, and environmental stimuli.[86–89] Poor sleep can exacerbate symptoms of cognitive function, fatigue, irritability, and difficulty concentrating, leading to significant morbidity, poor quality of life, and prolonged recovery. In 443 concussed patients with sleep-wake disturbances (SWD), Chaput and colleagues[90] found the patients were more likely to suffer from concomitant headaches, depressive symptoms, and irritability.

Conservative management begins with emphasis on sleep hygiene, including regular bedtime and rise time, avoiding stimulants and heavy exercise late in the day, limiting technology use before bed, avoiding spending time in bed awake, and improving sleep consolidation (ie, the ability to maintain sleep with minimal interruption).[91] Returning to daytime physical and mental activities also may be helpful in restoring sleep architecture.[92] Assessment for underlying psychiatric disorders should be performed, as anxiety and depression have been associated with greater daytime sleepiness, poorer sleep quality, and more naps in TBI versus controls.[93] In addition, any pain complaints should be evaluated and treated. If sleep disturbance is related to anxiety or other underlying psychiatric condition, referral to a behavioral health specialist for assistance with implementation of sleep hygiene and relaxation techniques can be considered.

Limited evidence exists regarding medication management of sleep disorders of TBI, and treatment strategies are adopted often from insomnia literature. Trazodone, a selective serotonin reuptake inhibitor (SSRI), has been used most commonly despite limited research regarding its efficacy. It has a favorable side-effect profile with anxiolytic and hypnotic properties.[92] Side effects can include dry mouth, dizziness, nausea, priapism, and headache.

Melatonin, an endogenous hormone produced by the pineal gland, also has a safe side-effect profile and may potentially be neuroprotective.[94,95] Although the exact mechanism of action is unclear, it is hypothesized to play a role in the regulation of circadian rhythm, reduction in core temperature, and via direct action on brain structures responsible for sleep.[92,96]

In a study of blast-related concussions in Iraq/Afghanistan veterans, prazosin, an alpha-1 antagonist, in combination with sleep hygiene counseling, compared with counseling alone demonstrated improvements in sleep, headaches, and cognition. This was felt to be secondary to prazosin's ability to decrease sleep latency and nocturnal arousals.[97]

Amitriptyline, a tricyclic antidepressant, can be considered in patients complaining of SWD in addition to posttraumatic headache and mood disorder and may be a desirable choice to avoid polypharmacy in patients with this multitude of symptoms. However, its use in concussion has not been well-studied and caution must be used in patients with cardiovascular disease, in geriatric patients, and in women of childbearing age.

Although benzodiazepines are effective in inducing sleep and reducing anxiety, they have been shown to be potentially detrimental to neurorecovery and should be used with caution.[98] Nonbenzodiazepine hypnotics, including zolpidem, can be considered; however, potential side effects in TBI are unknown and these medications should be used in low doses to reduce the risk of adverse effects. Somnambulation and cognitive impairment have been described.

Headache

Posttraumatic headache (PTH) is the most commonly reported symptom after concussion. Prevalence of PTH has been found to range from 30% to 90%, with 18% to 22% lasting more than 1 year.[99] PTH is typically classified as a secondary headache disorder and is diagnosed based on its close temporal relationship to injury (onset within 7 days). The most commonly reported headache types are migraine/probable migraine, tension, and cervicogenic when classified using The International Classification of Headache Disorders (ICHD)-2 diagnostic criteria.[100] Other variables related to trauma may complicate the diagnosis, such as medication overuse, emotional distress, myofascial pain, occipital neuralgia, cervical referred pain, and vascular etiologies. Whiplash injury occurs as a result of excessive neck extension-flexion secondary to acceleration-deceleration forces, and myofascial pain is a predominant feature. Myofascial injury may lead to tension-type headaches. Additionally, neuralgic headache pain may result from injuries to the occipital nerves or facet joints. Previous history of primary headache disorder and female gender have been described as risk factors for development of PTH.[101]

History should include headache location, pain characteristics, frequency, duration, severity, associated symptoms (such as nausea, vomiting, photo/phonosensitivity), and any aggravating/alleviating factors. Of note, headache characteristics may change from headache to headache or as time from initial injury passes. Patients also may present with characteristics of more than one subtype of headache. Migraine typically presents as a unilateral, moderate to severe, throbbing headache that worsens with activity and is accompanied by nausea, vomiting, and photophobia and/or phonophobia. Tension-type headache is characterized by mild to moderate bilateral pain that is viselike in nature, does not worsen with activity, and has no systemic systems, such as nausea, vomiting, or light and/or sound sensitivity.

Initial management should include education regarding proper sleep hygiene, exercise, and dietary considerations. Common headache triggers include irregular eating schedules, dehydration, too much or too little sleep, and reduced physical activity. Should there be a relationship between cognitive exertion and headache, interventions such as rest breaks during the day and school/work accommodations may be helpful.

Biologically based interventions include a variety of biofeedback mechanisms, physical therapy, manual therapy, immobilization devices, ice, and injections. Using systematic review, Wantabe and colleagues[102] found a single class II study in which manual spine therapy was found to be superior to treatment with cold packs alone in patients with PTH after concussion. However, treatment effect was not sustained past 8 weeks.[103] Three class III studies provided evidence for utilization of cognitive and/or behavioral therapy, biofeedback, and relaxation techniques for treatment of PTH; however, Tatrow and colleagues[104] found no statistically significant differences between types of treatments.[105,106] In a case series by Hect,[107] 8 of 10 patients with mixed TBI severity experienced complete relief of occipital neuralgia pain following 5% bupivacaine blocks. Finally, for treatment of whiplash injury, active therapy versus immobilization in a cervical collar demonstrated a lower percentage of patients with headaches in the therapy group.[108] Freund and Schwartz[109] also found patients who received onabotulinum toxin A for whiplash injury fared significantly better at 2 and 4 weeks than patients who received saline injections.

Pharmacologic treatment approach to PTH is twofold: acute or abortive therapy used on an as-needed basis and preventive therapy or prophylaxis used on a daily basis when attack frequency is high or patients fail to respond adequately to acute therapy interventions.[110] Nonspecific acute therapies, such as aspirin, acetaminophen, paracetamol, and nonsteroidal anti-inflammatory drugs, are generally less effective than more specific acute therapies; however, they may be helpful if used early when pain is mild and symptoms are developing slowly.[110] Potential side effects include gastritis, gastrointestinal bleeding, increased bleeding time, and peptic ulcer disease. Frequent use of these medications may contribute to rebound headaches and it is recommended that their use be limited to no more than 3 times per week. Specific acute therapies for migrainous symptoms include triptans, ergotamines, and dihydroergotamine (DHE), which are primarily serotonin 1B/D agonists. With the development of triptans, ergots are being used less frequently due to poor absorption and nausea when taken orally. Triptans possess vasoconstrictive properties and are contraindicated in patients with vascular disease. Finally, DHE is available in a nasal form, which has inconsistent absorption, or an injectable form, which is inconvenient to use.[100] Use of opioids for treatment of PTH is not recommended given the relative ineffectiveness for migraine phenotypes, risk of dependency and overuse, and sedating effects that may impair cognitive function.[100,111]

Preventive treatment may be considered when use of abortive medications fails to control frequency or intensity of attacks, pain is disabling, and there is concern for medication overuse. Preventive treatments have been shown to decrease headache frequency, severity, and duration and may improve the response to acute therapies.[110] The only medications that have been approved by the Food and Drug Administration for use in migraine are propranolol, timolol, valproic acid, and topiramate. Amitriptyline and topiramate have been found to be effective in treatment of tension-type headache in patients without concussion.[112,113] SSRIs and selective norepinephrine reuptake inhibitors are also used but less commonly. Patients also may find herbal, vitamin, and mineral supplements helpful.[100] Supplementation with magnesium, vitamin B2, alpha lipoic acid, and coenzyme q10 have been found to be effective in randomized double-blinded studies; however, their use has not been studied specifically for treatment of PTH.[114-117] The mechanism of action of preventive therapies is unknown; however, hypotheses include inhibition of cortical spreading depression, inhibition of glutamate dependent mechanisms, and modulation of serotonergic, dopaminergic, and adrenergic pathways and receptors.[100] Beta blockers decrease vascular dilation, and prevent platelet adhesion and aggregation while reducing the central activity of catecholamines.[118] Anticonvulsants facilitate neuronal inhibition via GABA potentiation while reducing neuronal hyperexcitability,[119] and tricyclic antidepressants (TCAs) alter central monamines, specifically serotonin.[118]

Vestibular/Vision Dysfunction

Together, the vestibular, oculomotor, and somatosensory systems consist of highly specialized neural networks with direct, indirect, and reciprocal projections to the spinal cord, autonomic nervous system, brainstem nuclei, cerebellum, thalamus, basal ganglia, and cerebral cortex.[120] Through special sensory organs located within the vestibulum of the inner ear, skin, muscles, joints, and brainstem, they interact to regulate gait, maintain balance and postural control, and coordinate eye movements. The VOR regulates gaze stabilization during head acceleration and the vestibulo-spinal reflex coordinates head, neck, and trunk positioning during dynamic body movements. Dysfunction within these components may adversely affect subsystems, leading to complex symptoms and impairments. Dizziness has been correlated with other PCS symptoms, particularly headache and anxiety.[121,122]

Dizziness and postural instability have been reported in up to 80% in the days to weeks following concussion. Causes have been found to be both central and peripheral in nature and include posttraumatic benign paroxysmal positional vertigo, labyrinth concussion, perilymphatic fistula, endolymphatic hydrops, otolith disorders, and central vestibulopathy; 46% of patients have been found to have dysfunction related to more than one mechanism.[121,123-127]

Patients will often complain of diplopia or blurry vision, convergence deficiencies with difficulty reading (such as losing their spot or skipping words), eye strain, motion sensitivity, or difficulty walking on uneven surfaces, headache, and anxiety in crowded places.[128,129] The physical examination should involve testing of visual acuity and visual fields, pupillary function, extraocular movements, convergence, and vergence. Often symptoms of dizziness, headache, and blurred vision will be elicited, and it is important to document which tests provoke symptoms. Mucha and colleagues[130] conducted a cross-sectional study for validity using the Vestibular-Ocular Motor Screen (VOMS), a brief clinical screening tool used to assess vestibular/ocular motor impairments and symptoms of sports-related concussions. The VOMS demonstrated internal consistency as well as sensitivity in identifying patients (n = 64) with concussions based on correlations with the Post Concussion Symptom Scale. Patients were tested between 0.5 and 9.5 days after concussion, and although the role of VOMS testing in PCS is unclear, it may be a useful tool for diagnosis of vestibular/oculomotor impairments.

Vestibular therapy and repositioning techniques are the cornerstones of treatment and have been demonstrated to be helpful after concussion.[127,131,132] Principles of vestibular rehabilitation include recalibration of depth and spatial perception under static and dynamic conditions by reestablishing efficient integration of the vestibular, visual, and somatosensory subsystems.[133] Treatment programs should be designed to improve function of the VOR, cervico-ocular reflex, depth perception, somatosensory retraining, dynamic gait, and aerobic training.[134]

Vision therapy programs for oculomotor dysfunction (OD) following concussion are also supported in the literature.[134] In a study of 160 patients with TBI, 90% demonstrated improvement of OD after completing vision therapy.[135] Vision therapy programs consist of exercises to improve function with fixation, pursuit, predictable and unpredictable saccade, mergence, and accommodation.[133]

Finally, should symptoms limit participation in therapies or significantly affect quality of life, a trial of vestibular suppressants (ie, meclizine) for peripheral causes or anxiolytics (ie, clonazepam) for central causes can be considered. Use of vestibular suppressants following concussion has not been studied, and efficacy is unknown. Additionally, use of vestibular suppressants may limit the brain's ability to compensate for centrally driven vestibular disorders.

Emotional

Although most concussion symptoms will improve with education, reassurance, healthy coping strategies, and the support of family and friends, persistent symptoms may be secondary to an interaction of pathophysiological and psychological etiologies. Prolonged cognitive, sleep, and somatic symptoms may result in patients becoming frustrated or anxious. Patients also may feel increasingly isolated as a result of treatment (physical and cognitive rest) that imposes limitations on activities such as school, work, and athletics. Emotional symptoms may contribute to the expression or persistence of PCS. Perceptions of physical symptoms may be exacerbated, and if emotional symptoms are left untreated, they can mimic neurocognitive symptoms of concussion. History of preexisting psychiatric disorders should be established, as premorbid depression and anxiety are known risk factors for the development of PCS.[31,136]

Cognitive behavioral therapy (CBT) is recommended as an overall first-line treatment for anxiety and depressive reactions. CBT aims to improve self-esteem, problem-solving skills, and psychosocial functioning following TBI and decreases depressive, anxiety, or anger symptoms. Behavioral interventions also may reduce the frequency of problematic behaviors or cognitive distortions resulting from injury that may prolong recovery.[75]

If emotional symptoms are persistent despite conservative interventions, pharmacologic treatment should be considered. SSRIs are often used as a first-line pharmacologic intervention in this population, and agents with no antimuscarinic effects are preferred, as this can impair cognitive function.[92] Sertraline, citalopram, or escitalopram have been shown to be effective for treating depressive symptoms, self-reported postconcussive symptoms, and cognition.[128–139] Paroxetine has been found to be as effective as citalopram at treating emotional symptoms in concussion; however, it does possess antimuscarinic properties and should be used with caution.[140,141] Fluoxetine also has been considered and is generally well tolerated; however, it has the potential for drug-drug interactions given its significant cytochrome P450 inhibition.[141] With TCAs, although considered effective for other symptoms of PCS, such as posttraumatic headaches and sleep dysfunction, evidence for efficacy in TBI-related depression is lacking.[142] All psychotropic medications should be used with caution in the adolescent population, as they can increase risk of suicidality.[143] Parental consent and close monitoring are warranted.

Cognitive

It has been reported that 40% to 60% of patients with TBI experience cognitive impairment at 1 to 3 months after injury.[142] Symptoms may include impaired memory, concentration, processing speed, and mental "fogginess," which may lead to declining academic or work performance. Patients also may report worsening somatic symptoms with cognitive exertion. Underlying factors such as emotional symptoms, sleep disturbance, chronic pain, or medication side effects should be evaluated. Neuropsychological testing can be helpful in assessing cognitive deficits in a quantitative manner.

Although most cognitive symptoms resolve over time, in those with significantly protracted recovery, cognitive rehabilitation may be helpful to develop compensatory strategies for cognitive deficits. For example, use of memory logs, to-do lists, and digital alarms set with reminders may help with memory and organization. Portable mobile electronic devices contain most of these features in a compact form and use should be encouraged. Cicerone and colleagues[144,145] and Rohling and colleagues[146] have established efficacy of cognitive rehabilitation in both civilian and military populations. Referral to speech therapies may be appropriate for individuals who experience adverse effects on work or school performance due to cognitive difficulties.

Evidence supporting the use of neurostimulants for treatment of cognitive deficits after TBI is emerging. This is based on the understanding of the biological effects of neurotransmitters on the regulation of cognitive activity; however, there are no randomized controlled studies and this has been identified as an area of needed study.

Dopamine, a neurotransmitter involved in the transmission of signals linked to executive function, arousal, and memory, has been targeted for its neurorecovery potential. Dopaminergic agonists are frequently used to address cognitive impairment following TBI.[147] In a study of concussed adolescent athletes, use of amantadine was associated with improvements in verbal memory and reaction time on computerized neurocognitive testing, as well as improvements in reported symptoms.[148] Giacino and colleagues[149] found amantadine accelerated the pace of functional recovery in 184 vegetative or minimally conscious patients during active treatment 4 to 16 weeks after injury compared with placebo. Amantadine increases the concentration of dopamine in the synaptic cleft through both presynaptic and postsynaptic actions. Additionally, it acts as an antagonist at N-methyl-D-aspartate (glutamate) receptors and may be neuroprotective.[150,151] This medication is generally well tolerated and common side effects include gastrointestinal complaints (diarrhea, constipation, nausea), orthostatic hypotension, and increased irritability. Livedo reticularis, a lacelike purplish discoloration of the skin, may be observed and can become permanent. Use with caution in those with a previous history of compulsive behaviors, as amantadine can worsen these.

Medications used in the treatment of attention-deficit disorder and attention-deficit/hyperactivity disorder that target both dopamine and norepinephrine through presynaptic and postsynaptic mechanisms have also been considered in the treatment of cognitive impairment following TBI. Randomized studies using methylphenidate in moderate to severe TBI showed improvement of attention deficits and processing speed.[152,153] However, no randomized-placebo controls exist. Side effects of these medications include elevated heart rate and blood pressure in higher doses and should be used with caution, if at all, in people with cardiac abnormalities (arrhythmias, recent myocardial infarction, structural abnormalities, cardiomyopathy, severe cardiac disease). Additionally, patients with history of motor tics/Tourette syndrome may experience tic worsening. Finally, cholinergic agents, such as donepezil, a long-acting acetylcholinesterase inhibitor, has been shown to improve short-term and long-term memory in patients with TBI.[92]

SUMMARY

Most individuals who experience concussion can expect full recoveries within the weeks to months after injury; however, some may have a more prolonged recovery course. It is clear from the literature that treatment approaches for this patient subset must be individualized. Clinicians managing this population should be skilled in the evaluation of overlapping symptoms and underlying contributing factors, patient education and reassurance, and use of nonpharmacologic and pharmacologic treatments when necessary.

REFERENCES

1. Aubry M, Cantu R, Dvorak J, et al. Summary and agreement statement of the 1st International Symposium on Concussion in Sport, Vienna 2001. Clin J Sport Med 2002;12:6–11.
2. McCrory P, Meeuwisse W, Johnston K, et al. Consensus statement on concussion in sport: the 3rd International Conference on Concussion in Sport held in Zurich, November 2008. Br J Sports Med 2009;43:176–84.
3. McCrory P, Johnston K, Meeuwisse W, et al. Summary and agreement statement of the 2nd International Conference on Concussion in Sport, Prague 2004. Br J Sports Med 2005;39:196–204.
4. McCrory P, Meeuwisse WH, Aury M, et al. Consensus statement on concussion in sport: the 4th International Conference on Concussion in Sport held in Zurich, November 2012. Br J Sports Med 2013;47:250–8.
5. Babcock L, Byczkowski T, Wade SL, et al. Predicting postconcussion syndrome after mild traumatic brain injury in children and adolescents who present to the emergency department. JAMA Pediatr 2013;167:156–61.
6. Chrisman SP, Rivara FP, Schiff MA, et al. Risk factors for concussive symptoms 1 week or longer in high school athletes. Brain Inj 2013;27:1–9.
7. Eisenberg MA, Andrea J, Meehan W, et al. Time interval between concussions and symptom duration. Pediatrics 2013;132:8–17.
8. McCrory PR, Ariens M, Berkovic SF. The nature and duration of acute concussive symptoms in Australian football. Clin J Sport Med 2000;10:235–8.
9. Erlanger D, Kaushik T, Cantu R, et al. Symptom based assessment of the severity of a concussion. J Neurosurg 2003;98:477–84.
10. Benson BW, Meeuwisse WH, Rizos J, et al. A prospective study of concussions among National Hockey League players during regular season games: the NHL-NHLPA Concussion Program. Can Med Assoc J 2011;183:905–11.
11. McCrea M, Guskiewicz KM, Marshall SW, et al. Acute effects and recovery time following concussion in collegiate football players – the NCAA Concussion Study. JAMA 2003;290:2556–63.
12. Lovell MR, Collins MW, Iverson GL, et al. Recovery from mild concussion in high school athletes. J Neurosurg 2003;98:296–301.
13. Makdissi M, Darby D, Maruff P, et al. Natural history of concussion in sport: markers of severity and implications for management. Am J Sports Med 2010; 38:464–71.
14. Rose S, Fischer A, Heyer G. How long is too long? The lack of consensus regarding the post-concussion syndrome diagnosis. Brain Inj 2015;29(7–8): 798–803.
15. Lees-Haley PR, Brown RS. Neuropsychological complaint base rates of 170 personal injury claimants. Arch Clin Neuropsychol 1993;8:203–9.

16. Iverson GL, McCracken LM. 'Postconcussive' symptoms in persons with chronic pain. Brain Inj 1997;11:783–90.
17. Mickeviciene D, Schrader H, Obelieniene D, et al. A controlled prospective inception cohort study on the post-concussion syndrome outside the medico-legal context. Eur J Neurol 2004;11:411–9.
18. Cooper DB, Kennedy JE, Cullen MA, et al. Association between combat stress and post-concussive symptom reporting in OEF/OIF service members with mild traumatic brain injuries. Brain Inj 2011;25:1–7.
19. Iverson GL. Misdiagnosis of the persistent postconcussion syndrome in patients with depression. Arch Clin Neuropsychol 2006;21:303–10.
20. Giza C, Hovda D. The neurometabolic cascade of concussion. J Athl Train 2001; 36(3):228–35.
21. Wu A, Ying Z, Gomez-Pinilla F. Vitamin E protects against oxidative damage and learning disability after mild TBI in rats. Neurorehabil Neural Repair 2010;24: 290–8.
22. Rathbone A, Tharmaradinam S, Jiang S, et al. A review of the neuro- and systemic inflammatory responses in post concussion symptoms: introduction of the "post-inflammatory brain syndrome" PIBS. Brain Behav Immun 2015;46: 1–16.
23. Kabadi SV, Stoica BA, Loane DJ, et al. CR8, a novel inhibitor of CDK, limits microglial activation, astrocytosis, neuronal loss, and neurologic dysfunction after experimental traumatic brain injury. J Cereb Blood Flow Metab 2014;34(3): 502–13.
24. Maroon JC, LePere DB, Blaylock RL, et al. Postconcussion syndrome: a review of pathophysiology and potential nonpharmacological approaches to treatment. Phys Sportsmed 2012;40(4):73–87.
25. Giza CC, Kutcher JS, Ashwal S, et al. Summary of evidence based guideline update: evaluation and management of concussion in sports: report of the Guideline Development Subcommittee of the American Academy of Neurology. Neurology 2013;80(24):2250–7.
26. Henry LC, Elbin RJ, Collins MW, et al. Examining recovery trajectories after sport-related concussion with a multimodal clinical assessment approach. Neurosurgery 2016;78(2):232–41.
27. Kay T, Newman B, Cavallo M, et al. Toward a neuropsychological model of functional disability after mild traumatic brain injury. Neuropsychology 1992;6: 371–84.
28. Meares S, Shores EA, Taylor AJ, et al. The prospective course of postconcussion syndrome: the role of mild traumatic brain injury. Neuropsychology 2011; 25:454–65.
29. Fox DD, Lees-Haley PR, Ernest K, et al. Post-concussive symptoms: base rates and etiology in psychiatric patients. Clin Neuropsychol 1995;9:89–92.
30. Evered L, Ruff R, Baldo J, et al. Emotional risk factors and postconcussional disorder. Assessment 2003;10:420–7.
31. Hou R, Moss-Morris R, Peveler R, et al. When a minor head injury results in enduring symptoms: a prospective investigation of risk factors for postconcussional syndrome after mild traumatic brain injury. J Neurol Neurosurg Psychiatry 2012;83:217–23.
32. Kutcher J, Eckner JT. At risk populations in sports related concussion. Curr Sports Med Rep 2010;9:16–20.
33. Finnoff JT, Jelsing EJ, Smith J. Biomarkers, genetics, and risk factors for concussion. PMR 2011;3:S452–9.

34. Cantu RC. Posttraumatic retrograde and anterograde amnesia: pathophysiology and implications in grading and safe return to play. J Athl Train 2001; 36:244–8.

35. Collins MW, Iverson GL, Lovell MR, et al. On field predictors of neuropsychological and symptom deficit following sports related concussion. Clin J Sport Med 2003;13:222–9.

36. Lau BC, Kontos AP, Collins MW, et al. Which on field signs/symptoms predict protracted recovery from sport related concussion among high school football players? Am J Sports Med 2011;39(11):2311-8.

37. Dischinger PC, Rybe GE, Kufera JA, et al. Early predictors of postconcussive syndrome in a population of trauma patients with mild traumatic brain injury. J Trauma 2009;66:289–96.

38. Dick RW. Is there a gender difference in concussion incidence and outcomes? Br J Sports Med 2009;43:146–50.

39. McCauley SR, Boake C, Levin HS, et al. Postconcussional disorder following mild to moderate traumatic brain injury: anxiety, depression and social support as risk factors and comorbidities. J Clin Exp Neuropsychol 2001;23:792–808.

40. Farace E, Alves WM. Do women fare worse? A metaanalysis of gender differences in outcome after traumatic brain injury. Neurosurg Focus 2000;8:e6.

41. Colvin AC, Mullen J, Lovell ME, et al. The role of concussion history and gender in recovery from soccer-related concussion. Am J Sports Med 2009;37: 1699–704.

42. Guskiewicz KM, McCrea M, Marshall SW, et al. Cumulative effects associated with recurrent concussion in collegiate football players: the NCAA Concussion Study. J Am Med Assoc 2003;290:2549–55.

43. Collins MW, Lovell MR, Iverson GL, et al. Cumulative effects of concussion in high school athletes. Neurosugery 2002;51:1175–9.

44. Slobounov S, Slobounov E, Sebastianelli W, et al. Differential rate of recovery in athletes after first and second concussion episodes. Neurosurgery 2007;61: 338–44.

45. Collins MW, Grindel SH, Lovell MR, et al. Relationship between concussion and neuropsychological performance in college football players. JAMA 1999;282: 964–70.

46. Moser RS, Schatz P, Jordan BD. Prolonged effects of concussion in high school athletes. Neurosurgery 2005;57:300–6.

47. Collie A, McCrory P, Makdissi M. Does history of concussion affect current cognitive status? Br J Sports Med 2006;40:802–5.

48. Straume-Naesheim TM, Anderson TE, Dvorak J, et al. Effects of heading exposure and previous concussions on neuropsychological performance among Norwegian elite footballers. Br J Sports Med 2005;39(Suppl 1):i70–7.

49. Wenham P, Price WH, Blundell G. Apolipoprotein E genotyping by one stage PCR. Lancet 1991;337:1158–9.

50. Lynch JR, Pineda JA, Morgan D, et al. Apolipoprotein E affects the central nervous system response to injury and the development of cerebral edema. Ann Neurol 2002;51:113–7.

51. Lucotte G, Visvikis S, Leininger M, et al. Association of apolipoprotein E allele epsilon 4 with late onset sporadic Alzheimer's disease. Am J Med Genet 1994;54:286–8.

52. Teasdale GM, Nicoll JA, Murray G, et al. Association of apolipoprotein E polymorphism with outcome after head injury. Lancet 1997;350:1069–71.

53. Friedman G, Froom P, Sazbon L. Apolipoprotein E epsilon 4 genotype predicts poor outcome in survivors of traumatic brain injury. Neurology 1999;53:244–8.

54. Kristman VL, Tator CH, Kreiger N, et al. Does the apolipoprotein epsilon 4 allele predispose varsity athletes to concussion? A prospective cohort study. Clin J Sport Med 2008;18:322–8.

55. Chamelian L, Reis M, Feinstein A. Six month recovery from mild to moderate traumatic brain injury: the role of APOE epsilon 4 allele. Brain 2004;127(Pt 12):2621–8.

56. Pruthi N, Chandramouli BA, Kuttappa TB, et al. Apolipoprotein E polymorphism and outcome after mild to moderate traumatic brain injury: a study of patient population in India. Neurol India 2010;58:264–9.

57. Terrell TR, Bostick RM, Abramson R, et al. APOE, APOE promoter and tau genotypes and risk for concussion in college athletes. Clin J Sport Med 2008; 18:10–7.

58. Schneider RC. Head and neck injuries in football: mechanisms, treatment and prevention. Baltimore (MD): Williams & Wilkins; 1973.

59. Iverson GL, Brooks BL, Lovell MR, et al. No cumulative effects for one or two previous concussions. Br J Sports Med 2006;40:72–5.

60. Bruce JM, Echemendia RJ. History of multiple self-reported concussions is not associated with reduced cognitive abilities. Neurosurgery 2009;64:100–6.

61. Matser EJ, Kessels AG, Lezak MD, et al. Neuropsychological impairment in amateur soccer players. JAMA 1999;282:971–3.

62. Matser EJ, Kessels AG, Lezak MD, et al. Chronic traumatic brain injury in professional soccer players. Neurology 1998;51:791–6.

63. Wall SE, Williams WH, Cartwright-Hatton S, et al. Neuropsychological dysfunction following repeat concussions in jockeys. J Neurol Neurosurg Psychiatry 2006;77:518–20.

64. DeBeaumont L, Theoret H, Mongeon D, et al. Brain function decline in healthy retired athletes who sustained their last sports concussion in early adulthood. Brain 2009;132:695–708.

65. DeBeaumont L, Brisson B, Lassonde M, et al. Long term electrophysiological changes in athletes with a history of multiple concussions. Brain 2007;21: 631–44.

66. Gaetz M, Goodman D, Weinberg H. Electrophysiological evidence for the cumulative effects of concussion. Brain Inj 2000;14:1077–88.

67. Theriault M, DeBeaumont L, Tremblay S, et al. Cumulative effects of concussions in athletes revealed by electrophysiological abnormalities on visual working memory. J Clin Exp Neuropsychol 2010;17:1–12.

68. Guskiewicz KM, Marshall SW, Bailes J, et al. Association between recurrent concussion and late life cognitive impairment in retired professional football players. Neurosurgery 2005;57:719–26.

69. DeBeaumont L, Henry LC, Gosselin N. Long term functional alterations in sports concussion. Neurosurg Focus 2012;33(6):E8.

70. Zhang L, Ravdin LD, Relkin N, et al. Increased diffusion in the brain of professional boxers: a preclinical sign of traumatic brain injury? AJNR Am J Neuroradiol 2003;24:52–7.

71. McKee AC, Cantu RC, Nowinski CJ, et al. Chronic traumatic encephalopathy in athletes: progressive tauopathy after repetitive head injury. J Neuropathol Exp Neurol 2009;68:709–35.

72. Jordan BD, Jahre C, Hauser WA, et al. CT of 338 active professional boxers. Radiology 1992;185:509–12.

73. Cantu RC. When to disqualify an athlete after a concussion. Curr Sports Med Rep 2009;8:6–7.

74. Conder R, Conder AA. Neuropsychological and psychological rehabilitation interventions in refractory sport-related post concussive syndrome. Brain Inj 2015; 29(2):249–62.

75. Marshall S, Bayley M, McCullagh S, et al. Updated clinical practice guidelines for concussion/mild traumatic brain injury and persistent symptoms. Brain Inj 2015;29(6):688–700.

76. Dacey RG, Alves WM, Rimel RW, et al. Neurosurgical complications after apparently minor head injury. Assessment of risk in a series of 610 patients. J Neurosurg 1986;65:203–10.

77. Kuppermann N. Pediatric head trauma: the evidence regarding indications for emergent neuroimaging. Pediatr Radiol 2008;38(Suppl 4):S670–4.

78. Gonzalez PG, Walker MT. Imaging modalities in mild traumatic brain injury and sports concussion. PMR 2011;3:S413–24.

79. Johnston KM, McCrory P, Mohtadi NG, et al. Evidence based review of sport related concussion: clinical science. Clin J Sport Med 2001;11:150–9.

80. Miller LJ, Mittenberg W. Brief cognitive behavioral interventions in mild traumatic brain injury. Appl Neuropsychol 1998;5:172–83.

81. Thomas DG, Apps JN, Hoffmann RG, et al. Benefits of strict rest after acute concussion: a randomized controlled trial. Pediatrics 2015;135:213–23.

82. DiFazio M, Siverberg ND, Kirkwood MW, et al. Prolonged activity restriction after concussion: are we worsening outcomes? Clin Pediatr (Phila) 2015. [Epub ahead of print].

83. Meehan WP III. Medical therapies for concussion. Clin Sports Med 2011;30:115–24.

84. Kontos AP, Elbin RJ, Schatz P, et al. A revised factor structure for the post-concussion symptom scale: baseline and postconcussion factors. Am J Sports Med 2012;40:2376–84.

85. Kempf J, Werth E, Kaiser PR, et al. Sleep wake disturbances 3 years after traumatic brain injury. J Neurol Neurosurg Psychiatry 2010;81:1402–5.

86. Ouellet MC, Savard J, Morin CM. Insomnia following traumatic brain injury: a review. Neurorehabil Neural Repair 2004;18:187–98.

87. Beetar JT, Guilmette TJ, Sparadeo FR. Sleep and pain complaints in symptomatic traumatic brain injury and neurologic populations. Arch Phys Med Rehabil 1996;77:1298–302.

88. Prigatano GP, Stahl ML, Orr WC, et al. Sleep and dreaming disturbances in closed head injury patients. J Neurol Neurosurg Psychiatry 1982;45:78–80.

89. Perlis ML, Artiola L, Giles DE. Sleep complaints in chronic postconcussion syndrome. Percept Mot Skills 1997;84:595–9.

90. Chaput G, Giguere JF, Chauny JM, et al. Relationship among subjective sleep complaints, headaches, and mood alterations following a mild traumatic brain injury. Sleep Med 2009;10(7):713–6.

91. Kashluba S, Paniak C, Casey JE. Persistent symptoms associated with factors identified by the WHO Task Force on Mild Traumatic Brain Injury. Clin Neuropsychol 2008;22:195–208.

92. Petraglia AL, Maroon JC, Bailes JE. From the field of play to the field of combat: a review of the pharmacological management of concussion. Neurosurgery 2012;70:1520–33.

93. Ponsford JL, Parcell DL, Sinclair KL, et al. Changes in sleep patterns following traumatic brain injury: a controlled study. Neurorehabil Neural Repair 2013; 27(7):613–21.
94. Samantaray S, Das A, Thakore NP, et al. Therapeutic potential of melatonin in traumatic central nervous system injury. J Pineal Res 2009;47:134–42.
95. Reiter RJ, Korkmaz A. Clinical aspects of melatonin. Saudi Med J 2008;29: 1537–47.
96. Rogers NL, Dinges DF, Kennaway DJ, et al. Potential action of melatonin in insomnia. Sleep 2003;26:1058–9.
97. Ruff RL, Ruff SS, Wang XF. Improving sleep: initial headache treatment in OIF/ OEF veterans with blast induced mild traumatic brain injury. J Rehabil Res Dev 2009;46:1071–84.
98. Rao V, Rollings P. Sleep disturbances following traumatic brain injury. Curr Treat Options Neurol 2002;4:77–87.
99. Lew HL, Lin PH, Fuh JL, et al. Characteristics and treatment of headache after traumatic brain injury. A focused review. Am J Phys Med Rehabil 2006;85: 619–27.
100. Lucas S. Characterization and management of headache after mild traumatic brain injury. In: Kobeissy FH, editor. Brain neurotrauma: molecular, neuropsychological, and rehabilitation aspects. Boca Raton (FL): CRC Press; 2015. p. 93–102.
101. Hoffman J, Lucas S, Dickmen S, et al. Natural history of headache following traumatic brain injury. J Neurotrauma 2011;28:1–8.
102. Wantabe TK, Bell KR, Walker WC, et al. Systematic review of interventions for post-traumatic headache. PM R 2012;4(2):129–40.
103. Jensen OK, Nielsen FF, Vosmar L. An open study comparing manual therapy with the use of cold packs in the treatment of post-traumatic headache. Cephalalgia 1990;10:241–50.
104. Tatrow K, Blanchard EB, Silverman DJ. Posttraumatic headache: an exploratory treatment study. Appl Psychophysiol Biofeedback 2003;28:267–78.
105. Gurr B, Coetzer B. The effectiveness of cognitive behavioral therapy for post traumatic headaches. Brain Inj 2005;19:481–91.
106. Hickling EJ, Blanchard EB, Schwartz SP, et al. Headaches and motor vehicle accidents: results of the psychological treatment of post-traumatic headache. Headache Q 1992;3:285–9.
107. Hect JS. Occipital nerve blocks in postconcussive headaches: a retrospective review and report of ten patients. J Head Trauma Rehabil 2004;19:58–71.
108. Bonk AD, Ferrari R, Giebel GD, et al. Prospective, randomized, controlled study of activity versus collar, and the natural history for whiplash injury, in Germany. J Musculoskelet Pain 2000;8:123–32.
109. Freund BJ, Schwartz M. Treatment of chronic cervical associated headache with botulinum toxin a: a pilot study. Headache 2000;20:231–6.
110. Silberstein SD. Practice parameter: evidence based guidelines for migraine headache (an evidence based review): report of the quality standards subcommittee of the American Academy of Neurology. Neurology 2000;55:754–62.
111. Ramadan N, Silberstein SD, Freitag FG, et al. Evidence based guidelines for migraine headache in the primary care setting: pharmacological management for prevention of migraine. Neurology 1999;55:754–62.
112. Bendtsen L, Mathew NT. Prophylactic pharmacotherapy of tension-type headache. In: Olesen J, Goadsby PJ, Ramadan N, et al, editors. The headaches. Philadelphia: Lippincott Williams Wilkins; 2005. p. 735–41.

113. Lampl C, Marecek S, May A, et al. A prospective, open label, long term study of the efficacy and tolerability of topiramate in the prophylaxis of chronic tension type headache. Cephalalgia 2006;26(10):1203–8.

114. Peikert A, Wilimzig C, Kohne-Volland R. Prophylaxis of migraine with oral magnesium: results from a prospective, multicenter, placebo controlled and double blind randomized study. Cephalalgia 1996;16:257–63.

115. Shoenen J, Jacquy J, Lenaerts M. Effectiveness of high dose riboflavin in migraine prophylaxis. A randomized controlled trial. Neurology 1998;50:466–70.

116. Sandor PS, DiClemente L, Coppola G, et al. Efficacy of coenzyme Q10 in migraine prophylaxis: a randomized controlled trial. Neurology 2005;64:713–5.

117. Magis D, Ambrosini A, Sandor PS, et al. A randomized double blind placebo controlled trial of thioctic acid in migraine prophylaxis. Headache 2007;47:52–7.

118. Bell KR, Kraus EE, Zasler ND. Medical management of posttraumatic headaches: pharmacological and physical treatment. J Head Trauma Rehabil 1999;14:34–48.

119. Lane JC, Arciniegas DB. Post traumatic headache. Curr Treat Options Neurol 2002;4:89–104.

120. Armstrong B, McNair P, Taylor D. Head and neck position sense. Sports Med 2008;38:101–17.

121. Register-Mihalik JK, Mihalik JP, Guskiewicz KM. Balance deficits after sports related concussion in individuals reporting posttraumatic headache. Neurosurgery 2008;63:76–80.

122. Guskiewicz KM. Assessment of postural stability following sport related concussion. Curr Sports Med Rep 2003;2:24–30.

123. Maskell F, Chiarelli P, Isles R. Dizziness after traumatic brain injury: overview and management in the clinical setting. Brain Inj 2006;20:293–305.

124. Cavanaugh JT, Guskiewicz KM, Giuliani C, et al. Detecting altered postural control after cerebral concussion in athletes with normal postural stability. Br J Sports Med 2005;39:805–11.

125. Guskiewicz KM. Balance assessment in the management of sport related concussion. Clin Sports Med 2011;30:89–102.

126. Guskiewicz KM. Postural stability assessment following concussion: one piece of the puzzle. Clin J Sport Med 2001;11:182–9.

127. Ernst A, Basta D, Seidl RO, et al. Management of posttraumatic vertigo. Otolaryngol Head Neck Surg 2005;132:554–8.

128. Kapoor N, Ciuffreda KJ. Vision disturbances following traumatic brain injury. Curr Treat Options Neurol 2002;4:271–80.

129. Kapoor N, Ciuffreda KJ, Han Y. Oculomotor rehabilitation in acquired brain injury: a case series. Arch Phys Med Rehabil 2004;85:1667–78.

130. Mucha A, Collins MW, Furman JM, et al. A brief vestibular/ocular motor screening (VOMS) assessment to evaluate concussions: preliminary findings. Am J Sports Med 2014;42(10):2479–86.

131. Alsalaheen BA, Mucha A, Morris LO, et al. Vestibular rehabilitation for dizziness and balance disorders after concussion. J Neurol Phys Ther 2010;34:87–93.

132. Gottshall KR, Hoffer ME. Tracking recovery of vestibular function in individuals with blast induced head trauma using vestibular visual cognitive interaction tests. J Neurol Phys Ther 2010;34:94–7.

133. Ellis MJ, Leddy JJ, Willer B. Physiological, vestibule-ocular and cervicogenic post-concussion disorders: an evidence based classification system with directions for treatment. Brain Inj 2015;29(2):238–48.

134. Balaban CD, Hoffer ME, Gottshall KR. Top down approach to vestibular compensation: translational lessons from vestibular rehabilitation. Brain Res 2012;1482:101–11.

135. Ciuffreda KJ, Rutner D, Kapoor N, et al. Vision therapy for oculomotor dysfunctions in acquired brain injury: a retrospective analysis. Optometry 2008;79: 18–22.

136. Covassin T, Elbin RJ, Larson E, et al. Sex and age differences in depression and baseline sport related concussion neurocognitive performance and symptoms. Clin J Sport Med 2012;22:98–104.

137. Fann JR, Uomoto JM, Katon WJ. Sertraline in the treatment of major depression following mild traumatic brain injury. J Neuropsychiatry Clin Neurosci 2000;12: 226–32.

138. Fann JR, Uomoto JM, Katon WJ. Cognitive improvement with treatment of depression following mild traumatic brain injury. Psychosomatics 2001;42: 48–54.

139. Rapoport MJ, Chan F, Lanctot K, et al. An open label study of citalopram for major depression following traumatic brain injury. J Psychopharmacol 2008;22: 860–4.

140. Muller U, Murai T, Bauer-Wittmund T, et al. Paroxetine versus citalopram treatment of pathological crying after brain injury. Brain Inj 1999;13:805–11.

141. Silver JM, McAllister TW, Arciniegas DB. Depression and cognitive complaints following mild traumatic brain injury. Am J Psychiatry 2009;166:653–61.

142. Warden DL, Warden B, McAllister TW, et al. Guidelines for the pharmacologic treatment of neurobehavioral sequelae of traumatic brain injury. J Neurotrauma 2006;23:1468–501.

143. Hammad TA, Laughren T, Racoosin J. Suicidality in pediatric patients treated with antidepressant drugs. Arch Gen Psychiatry 2006;63:332–9.

144. Cicerone KD, Dahlberg C, Malec JF, et al. Evidence based cognitive rehabilitation: updated review of literature from 1988 through 2002. Arch Phys Med Rehabil 2005;86:1681–92.

145. Cicerone KD, Langenbahn DM, Braden C, et al. Evidence based cognitive rehabilitation: updated review of the literature from 2003 through 2008. Arch Phys Med Rehabil 2011;92:519–30.

146. Rohling ML, Beverly B, Faust ME, et al. Effectiveness of cognitive rehabilitation following acquired brain injury: a meta-analytic re-examination of Cicerone et al.'s (2000, 2005) systematic reviews. Neuropsychology 2009;23:20–39.

147. Lercher K, Reddy CC. Treating prolonged symptoms of mild traumatic brain injury: neuropharmacology. Concussion. Prog Neurol Surg 2014;28:139–48.

148. Reddy CC, Collins MW, Lovell M, et al. Efficacy of amantadine treatment on symptoms and neurocognitive performance among adolescents following sports related concussion. J Head Trauma Rehabil 2013;28:260–5.

149. Giacino JT, Whyte J, Bagiella E, et al. Placebo controlled trial of Amantadine for severe traumatic brain injury. N Engl J Med 2012;366:819–26.

150. Zafonte RD, Lexell J, Cullen N. Possible applications for dopaminergic agents following traumatic brain injury: part 2. J Head Trauma Rehabil 2001;16:112–6.

151. Meythaler JM, Brunner RC, Johnson A, et al. Amantadine to improve neurorecovery in traumatic brain injury associated diffuse axonal injury: a pilot double blind randomized trial. J Head Trauma Rehabil 2002;17:300–13.

152. Whyte J, Hart T, Vaccaro M, et al. Effects of methylphenidate on attention deficits after traumatic brain injury: a multidimensional, randomized, controlled trial. Am J Phys Med Rehabil 2004;83:401–20.

153. Plenger PM, Dixon CE, Castillo CE, et al. Subacute methylphenidate treatment for moderate to moderately severe traumatic brain injury: a preliminary double blind placebo controlled study. Arch Phys Med Rehabil 1996;77: 536–40.

The Role of Neuropsychological Evaluation in the Clinical Management of Concussion

Amy K. Connery, PsyD[a],*, Robin L. Peterson, PhD[a],
David A. Baker, PsyD[a], Christopher Randolph, PhD[b],
Michael W. Kirkwood, PhD[a]

KEYWORDS

- Mild TBI • Postconcussion syndrome • Neuropsychological assessment
- Traumatic brain injury

KEY POINTS

- Because the etiology of persistent symptoms after concussion is often complex and multi-factorial, neuropsychologists are well-positioned to understand and help manage such symptomatology.
- When unexpected difficulties are apparent or recovery is not progressing as expected, neuropsychological evaluation can help to identify factors serving to prolong recovery.
- After neuropsychological evaluation, interventions specifically tailored to address factors that may be prolonging recovery can help to improve functioning and minimize distress.

INTRODUCTION

Although most people recover quickly and completely after a single, uncomplicated mild traumatic brain injury (TBI) or concussion, a minority of patients experience persistent postconcussive symptoms. The etiology of such symptomatology is often complex and multifactorial, involving both injury and noninjury factors. Neuropsychologists, who have expertise in development, psychology, and brain injury,

Financial Disclosure: The authors have no financial relationships to disclose.
Conflict of Interest: The authors have no conflicts of interest to disclose.
[a] Department of Physical Medicine & Rehabilitation, Children's Hospital Colorado, University of Colorado School of Medicine, Aurora, CO, USA; [b] Department of Neurology, Loyola University Medical Center, 2160 S, First Ave, Maywood, IL 60153, USA
* Corresponding author. Department of Rehabilitation Medicine, Children's Hospital Colorado, 13123 East 16th Avenue, Aurora, CO 80045.
E-mail address: amy.connery@childrenscolorado.org

are well-positioned to understand and help manage such symptomatology. As such, neuropsychological evaluation is now widely recognized as an important component in the clinical management of individuals who sustain concussive injuries.[1-3]

NATURAL CLINICAL HISTORY

To manage any clinical condition, a clear understanding of its natural clinical history is imperative. Methodologically sound studies have now converged to paint a picture of what can be considered the "typical" recovery after concussion. In the first hours to days after injury, the neurobehavioral effects can be impressive, with pronounced postconcussive symptomatology reported, as well as changes apparent on objective cognitive and balance tests.[4] Problems are typically self-limiting and resolve gradually for the majority of individuals in the initial days to weeks. When using objective performance-based tests, most methodologically rigorous studies fail to identify significant differences between concussed and control groups within 7 to 10 days in high school athletes[5] and older athletes and within 2 to 3 months in nonathlete children and adults.[6-11] In contrast, when examining outcomes using subjectively reported symptoms, a minority of patients display more persistent problems.[12]

RISK FACTORS FOR PROLONGED RECOVERY

Both injury and noninjury factors have been found to play a role in persistent symptomatology. In general, injury-related variables (ie, the direct neurologic effects of concussion) account for more variance in the first weeks after the injury, and non–injury-related variables account for more variance in subsequent periods.[13] One factor that has been found to increase the risk of persistent problems is more severe mild TBI, such as injury characterized by intracranial pathology or need for hospitalization.[14-18] However, the effect of injury-related factors tends to diminish over time,[19] and many "postconcussive" symptoms are not driven by injury-related neurologic factors.

One set of non–injury-related variables that account for persistent problems after concussion are personality factors, including how an individual responds to stressful events. Specific personality traits and coping strategies can affect how one might understand and respond to a concussive injury.[20] In both adults and children, ineffective coping can serve to maintain symptoms and make one vulnerable to a prolonged recovery.[21-23]

Many patients expect that they will experience postconcussive symptoms and will have prolonged symptoms after an injury occurs, a phenomenon characterized by Mittenberg and colleagues[24] as "expectation as etiology." This expectation of negative outcome then results in errors of attribution with regard to benign symptoms and events. For example, a simple lapse of attention may be attributed to the effects of a concussion, while disregarding preinjury functioning or normal inattention. Therefore, in some cases, it is the expectation that symptoms will be prolonged that causes the prolonged recovery.[25]

The "good old days" bias has been recognized as another factor that influences symptom report after concussion. Patients and caregivers may underestimate the level of past concerns and attribute any current concerns to the injury. This bias has been well-demonstrated in adults[26] and was recently found in many parents of children after concussion.[27]

Preexisting behavioral and learning problems,[28-30] family functioning,[31] and caregiver adjustment[19] have been all been shown to contribute additionally to the variance in rates of recovery and in the prediction of symptom outcomes. Comorbidities, such as posttraumatic stress disorder, pain, and mood problems, are also important to identify because the effects of these disorders can mimic postconcussive symptoms.[32,33] Lower levels of education and female gender have been shown to be associated with increased symptom reporting as well.[33–35]

Although "brain rest" has been widely recommended in recent years as a cornerstone of concussion management, recent studies have suggested that rest, particularly prolonged rest, may in fact exacerbate postconcussive symptoms and serve to prolong recovery.[36,37] Prolonged rest may result in increased anxiety and negative expectations for recovery, depression with withdrawal from typical daily activities, and physical deconditioning.[38]

Another important factor influencing symptom presentation after concussion is whether a patient is exaggerating or feigning problems.[10,39–42] Exaggeration or feigning of symptoms occurs much less frequently in sports-related populations than in the general population of mild TBI, because most athletes are motivated to recover and return to their sport.[5] However, in children and adolescents referred for persistent symptoms, the rate of feigning is similar between athletes and nonathletes (around 17%–18% in previous studies of our clinic sample).[43,44]

Relatedly, litigation status also has been shown to influence symptom presentation after concussion.[10,39,45] Litigation was a less frequent occurrence in the context of sport-related concussion historically when compared with general mild TBI patient populations.[5] However, there has been a recent proliferation of lawsuits related to concussion in professional sports and a subsequent increase in lawsuits at all levels of sport.[46]

CONSIDERATIONS IN CLINICAL NEUROPSYCHOLOGICAL EVALUATIONS

Several factors should be considered when planning how to integrate neuropsychological assessment into the clinical management of concussion. Important considerations include determining whether baseline testing will be implemented, if computerized tests will be used, and how validity tests will be incorporated. Although an in-depth discussion of these issues is beyond the scope of this paper, a brief discussion is presented.

Baseline Testing

The use of baseline testing with athletes has become increasingly widespread in recent years. Cognitive testing within a "baseline" model involves evaluating athletes before a season begins and then repeating the same testing if a concussion occurs. Baseline testing has been promoted as an effective tool to assist in determining when a person has made a complete recovery and can safely return to play. At first blush, baseline testing has considerable intuitive appeal. However, a number of statistical problems (eg, poor test–retest reliability of commonly used measures) exist.[47–49] Moreover, at present, no identified empirical data are available to demonstrate that baseline cognitive testing actually improves clinical outcomes or reduces any known risk associated with concussive injury.[50] Owing to the lack of clear evidence regarding the clinical utility of baseline testing, the most recent guidelines from the Zurich Concussion in Sport Conference concluded that there is insufficient evidence to recommend the widespread routine use of baseline testing, although neuropsychological testing was recognized as important in some cases.[3]

Computerized Testing

Computerized tests are most often used because of the practical advantages of test administration. However, the practical appeal of computerized tests should not dictate adoption, because psychometric and testing expertise are important when considering whether or not to incorporate computerized cognitive tests into a concussion management plan. A critical appreciation of the psychometric properties of a test is crucial, because poor test–retest reliability and poor sensitivity and specificity have been reported for many computerized tests, as discussed. Inadequate understanding of the psychometrics (and the natural clinical history of concussion) increases the risks for both false-positive errors (ie, classifying someone as impaired when she or he is not) and false-negative errors (ie, classifying someone as intact when she or he is not).[5,48,49,51–53] Because many factors can contribute to neuropsychological test performance, it is not sufficient to simply administer a test and interpret the results in isolation. No computerized test is diagnostic for concussion, and test results need to be interpreted by an examiner qualified to consider all potential contributing factors in understanding test results. This includes an understanding of neuropsychological concepts, psychometrics, test interpretation in the context of history and other data, and the dynamic biopsychosocial context in which postconcussive symptoms can occur.[54]

Validity Testing

Understanding symptoms as neurologically based or related to nonneurologic or noninjury factors has clear implications for clinical decision making and management. As mentioned, an important factor that influences symptom presentation and neuropsychological test results is whether a patient is exaggerating symptomatology, exerting insufficient effort, and/or feigning. Multiple studies of both children and adults have shown that these are not uncommon occurrences in the context of persistent postconcussive symptomatology, with base rates ranging from about 15% to 20% in pediatric clinical settings[44,55] to 40% to 50% or more in adult compensation-seeking settings.[41,56] If an examinee exerts insufficient effort or intentionally performs poorly on a neuropsychological examination, the broader test results and self-report should not be considered valid.[40,43,57,58]

Performance validity is assessed by the use of stand-alone and embedded tests that are designed to seem difficult but in actuality are quite easy and can be performed well with very little effort or ability. Multiple studies have demonstrated that performance on these tests is unrelated to pain, neurologic status, and cognitive abilities, except in the most extreme cases.[59–63] Therefore, when patients perform poorly on these tests, a nonneurologic or non–injury-related explanation for the low scores is likely. Evaluating validity in clinical practice and addressing concerns for invalid test performance with patients and families is addressed in detail elsewhere.[64,65]

TIMELINE FOR NEUROPSYCHOLOGICAL EVALUATION

McCrea and colleagues[66] examined various metaanalytic studies on the natural clinical history of concussion. Based on this analysis, the authors defined 3 time points in recovery: the acute period (from the time of injury to approximately 5 days after the injury), the subacute period (from approximately 5–30 days after the injury), and a chronic period (when symptoms persist beyond 30 days). Most patients can be expected to be symptomatic in the acute period, and patients are typically managed medically during this period. A brief cognitive screening has been found to be as sensitive to sport-related concussion as lengthier testing in the acute period,[67] and can be useful in guiding management decisions soon after injury. Several instruments have been developed for this purpose, with the Standardized Assessment of Concussion being one of the most commonly used in sport settings.[68] Because most people recover relatively quickly after concussion, more comprehensive neuropsychological evaluation is typically not indicated during the acute period.

In the face of persistent problems during the subacute period, a relatively abbreviated neuropsychological evaluation could be appropriate, one that is more extensive than a very brief cognitive screening, but less extensive than a traditional neuropsychological assessment. This is likely justifiable and cost effective, because it can help to identify reasons for problems, assist in the creation of an appropriate clinical management plan, and reduce the risk of prolonged patient distress or secondary psychosocial problems.

Because most studies have concluded that measurable neurocognitive deficits completely resolve within a matter of days to weeks after concussion, some might question the role of neuropsychological assessment in the chronic period. However, for those patients who have apparently not returned to their baseline level of functioning, a neuropsychological evaluation is likely worthwhile, to assist in identifying factors that may be producing problems, to ensure accurate diagnostic decisions have been made, and to help develop an appropriate clinical management plan. We recently completed a prospective, quasiexperimental study examining the value of neuropsychological evaluation during the chronic period and found evidence for substantially reduced postconcussive symptomatology after such consultation,[35] supporting the common clinical practice of referring for neuropsychological consultation in the face of persistent symptoms.

COMPONENTS OF NEUROPSYCHOLOGICAL EVALUATION

The following discussion is an adaption of a pediatric concussion neuropsychological management model proposed by Kirkwood and colleagues.[69] When conducting a neuropsychological evaluation, the neuropsychologist must first obtain a detailed injury history to establish that the patient did indeed suffer a concussion. Because concussion does not produce a diagnostically distinct cognitive or symptom profile, the diagnosis of concussion or determination of injury severity can never be based solely on neuropsychological testing or symptom ratings.[70–73] Therefore, the collection of injury-related information continues to be essential through interview and, whenever possible, objective records (eg, day of injury emergency transport or hospital records). In reviewing these data, careful consideration needs to be given to information that can be used to determine injury severity specifically. Injuries associated with a Glasgow Coma Scale score of lower than 13, neuroimaging abnormalities, a period of unconsciousness longer than 15 to 30 minutes, or posttraumatic amnesia longer than 24 hours could all suggest a more serious TBI, for which persistent problems might not be unexpected.

More comprehensive developmental, psychological/psychosocial, and educational/work information should also be gathered through interviews and objective records, to better understand the patient's preinjury functioning and to identify any factors that could be influencing postinjury presentation and neuropsychological test results (eg, premorbid attention or learning problems, psychiatric issues, family or work stressors). Because family factors can impact concussion recovery, family stressors and functioning should additionally be considered. Last, the patient and family's own expected course of recovery and litigation status need to be explored, because expectations and selective attentional biases after injury can have important effects on the concussion recovery process, as discussed.[24,27,74]

Assessment Instruments

It is reasonable to include a measure of postconcussive symptomatology in any postconcussion neuropsychological workup given that concussion has large effects on symptom experience acutely.[4] At the same time, the fact that "postconcussive" symptoms are nonspecific and can occur for innumerable reasons other than concussion must be kept in mind.[71,75,76] Assessment of performance within select cognitive domains will also be important. In general, processing speed and aspects of memory, attention, and executive functioning have demonstrated the most sensitivity to the effects of concussion.[10] Multiple batteries have been developed to examine these and related domains including both computerized and paper-and-pencil measures. Regardless of the instruments that are deemed most suitable for evaluating concussion effects, the results must be interpreted in the context of methodologically rigorous outcome studies demonstrating that the effects of concussion are typically small after the acute period and transient, as well as the technical weaknesses of the chosen instruments and limitations of using an abbreviated battery or test of any kind.

To facilitate proper interpretation, the postacute neuropsychological battery also should include coverage of domains that are likely to be insensitive to concussion. Most well-established or crystallized skills (eg, single word reading) should remain relatively preserved, even in the acute period after concussion. If performance on these measures is poor, consideration needs to be given to whether preinjury problems or other non–injury-related factors may be contributing to the findings.

To examine the contribution of psychological difficulties, personality or behavioral adjustment rating scales should be incorporated into the evaluation as well. Posttraumatic anxiety, pain, and sleep disturbance also need to be explicitly considered, because these are often associated with events that produce concussion (eg, motor vehicle collision). Studies with both adults and children suggest that these problems can affect neuropsychological and symptom presentation independent of the concussion.[77–82] During the chronic stage, broader based coverage of neurocognitive, psychosocial, and achievement functioning may be indicated, to allow for a complete picture of the patient's functional status and to help identify difficulties that may be contributing to persistent problems.

Neuropsychological Management Recommendations

Because there are a multitude of reasons patients may still be having difficulties months to years after a concussion, no generic management plan or treatment protocol is appropriate for all patients. Management recommendations need to be individually tailored and coordinated with other involved health care providers. Recommendations often include educational/work place accommodations soon after injury and other psychological/supportive approaches that help to address the individual's associated conditions as identified in the neuropsychological evaluation.[83] Continuing to provide education and reassurance is also appropriate months after injury, as is ensuring that reasonable attributions about the cause of symptoms have been developed. Patients and parents often underestimate their premorbid problems and thus can place too much emphasis on injury-related factors as the cause of their current symptoms.[24,84,85] Finally, minimal evidence exists that injury-focused therapies, such as cognitive remediation, are effective for concussion management.[86,87] In fact, injury-focused therapies may result in iatrogenesis in certain situations (eg, cases with a significant somatization component) and could serve to prolong recovery.

Return to Play

Although medical personnel ultimately decide on the safety of permitting participation in sports and other physical activity in most cases, the neuropsychological evaluation can assist in helping sort out the likely etiology of persistent symptoms to help guide return to play decisions. Activity restriction itself can have adverse effects on both mood and lifestyle, so athletes should be monitored closely when they are restricted from play.[88,89] Should concerns arise, referral to a sports psychologist or other behavioral health professional could be warranted. In the end, the return to play decision should rest on a careful, individualized, cost–benefit analysis weighing the potential risks of a return to sports with the psychosocial and other benefits of allowing a return to play.[90]

Pediatric Considerations

Soon after a pediatric concussion, school personnel should be notified of the injury, what to generally expect, the need to monitor the student for at least some days, and how best to support the student's recovery when the student comes back to school. This typically includes temporary and informal accommodations to help ensure children are supported adequately soon after injury. At the same time, students should be encouraged to return to school in a timely fashion, most often in a few days, given the potential iatrogenic effect removal from school can have. A number of resources have been developed for school personnel to help optimize this balance between proper understanding/support and reassurance and timely resumption of school activities (eg, Children's Hospital Colorado Return to Learn Program).[91]

In the context of persistent symptoms in the chronic phase, coordinating school-based supportive services with educators is often necessary. Whether supports are needed from an academic or psychosocial perspective (or both), documenting them in some type of informal or formal educational plan may be indicated (eg, 504 Plan). The nature of the educational plan will depend largely on the neuropsychological evaluation results, including a detailed characterization of the student's difficulties and an accurate determination of their likely etiology. Because concussion does not typically result in lasting academic problems, the educational plan should focus on the more likely non–injury-related etiology of the identified problems.

SUMMARY

Because the etiology of persistent symptoms after concussion is often complex and multifactorial, neuropsychological evaluation can be a useful intervention when a patient is not progressing as expected. Evaluation in the subacute (from approximately 5–30 days after the injury) and chronic periods (when symptoms persist beyond 30 days) can help to identify those factors that may be serving to prolong recovery and can assist in more specifically tailoring interventions to help improve functioning and minimize distress.

Although current assessment practice includes administration of tests measuring cognitive domains that are sensitive, as well as insensitive, to the effects of concussion, no single test battery has been shown to be superior over other batteries. Future studies are needed to compare different test batteries to determine which practices are most efficient and effective in postconcussion management.

Last, some medical practices and patients may not have access to a neuropsychologist and neuropsychological intervention. Future studies will also be needed to examine alternate means of service delivery to ensure that all patients with persistent postconcussive symptoms have access to this important component of care.

REFERENCES

1. Giza CC, Kutcher JS, Ashwal S, et al. Summary of evidence-based guideline update: evaluation and management of concussion in sports report of the Guideline

Development Subcommittee of the American Academy of Neurology. Neurology 2013;80:2250–7.

2. Harmon KG, Drezner JA, Gammons M, et al. American Medical Society for Sports Medicine position statement: concussion in sport. Br J Sports Med 2013;47: 15–26.

3. McCrory P, Davis G, Makdissi M. Second impact syndrome or cerebral swelling after sporting head injury. Curr Sports Med Rep 2012;11:21–3.

4. Broglio SP, Puetz TW. The effect of sport concussion on neurocognitive function, self-report symptoms and postural control: a meta-analysis. Sports Med 2008;38: 53–67.

5. Belanger HG, Vanderploeg RD. The neuropsychological impact of sports-related concussion: a meta-analysis. J Int Neuropsychol Soc 2005;11:345–57.

6. Babikian T, Asarnow R. Neurocognitive outcomes and recovery after pediatric TBI: meta-analytic review of the literature. Neuropsychology 2009;23:283–96.

7. Vu JA, Babikian T, Asarnow R. Academic and language outcomes in children and after traumatic brain injury. Except Child 2011;77:263–81.

8. Binder LM, Rohling ML, Larrabee GJ. A review of mild head trauma. Part I: meta-analytic review of neuropsychological studies. J Clin Exp Neuropsychol 1997;19: 421–31.

9. Schretlen DJ, Shapiro AM. A quantitative review of the effects of traumatic brain injury on cognitive functioning. Int Rev Psychiatry 2003;15:341–9.

10. Belanger HG, Curtiss G, Demery JA, et al. Factors moderating neuropsychological outcomes following mild traumatic brain injury: a meta-analysis. J Int Neuropsychol Soc 2005;11:215–27.

11. Rohling ML, Binder LM, Demakis GJ, et al. A meta-analysis of neuropsychological outcome after mild traumatic brain injury: re-analyses and reconsiderations of Binder et al. (1997), Frencham et al. (2005), and Pertab, et al. (2009). Clin Neuropsychol 2011;25:608–23.

12. Yeates KO, Taylor HG. Neurobehavioral outcomes. In: Kirkwood M, Yeates K, editors. Mild traumatic brain injury in children and adolescents: from basic science to clinical management. New York: Guilford Press; 2012. p. 124–41.

13. Iverson GL. Outcome from mild traumatic brain injury. Curr Opin Psychiatry 2005; 18:301–17.

14. Babcock L, Byczkowski T, Wade SL, et al. Predicting postconcussion syndrome after mild traumatic brain injury in children and adolescents who present to the emergency department. JAMA Pediatr 2013;167:156–61.

15. Barlow KM, Crawford S, Stevenson A, et al. Epidemiology of postconcussion syndrome in pediatric mild traumatic brain injury. Pediatrics 2010;126:e374–81.

16. Levin HS, Hanten G, Roberson G, et al. Prediction of cognitive sequelae based on abnormal computed tomography findings in children following mild traumatic brain injury. J Neurosurg Pediatr 2008;1:461–70.

17. Williams DH, Levin HS, Eisenberg HM. Mild head injury classification. Neurosurgery 1990;27:422–8.

18. Yeates KO, Taylor HG, Rusin J, et al. Premorbid child and family functioning as predictors of post-concussive symptoms in children with mild traumatic brain injuries. Int J Dev Neurosci 2012;30:231–7.

19. McNally KA, Bangert B, Dietrich A, et al. Injury versus noninjury factors as predictors of postconcussive symptoms following mild traumatic brain injury in children. Neuropsychology 2013;27:1–12.

20. Kay T. Neuropsychological treatment of mild traumatic brain injury. J Head Trauma Rehabil 1993;8:74–85.

21. Belanger HG, Barwick FH, Kip KE, et al. Postconcussive symptom complaints and potentially malleable positive predictors. Clin Neuropsychol 2013;27:343–55.
22. Iverson GL. Mild traumatic brain injury meta-analyses can obscure individual differences. Brain Inj 2010;24:1246–55.
23. Woodrome SE, Yeates KO, Taylor HG, et al. Coping strategies as a predictor of post-concussive symptoms in children with mild traumatic brain injury versus mild orthopedic injury. J Int Neuropsychol Soc 2011;17:317–26.
24. Mittenberg W, DiGiulio DV, Perrin S, et al. Symptoms following mild head injury: expectation as aetiology. J Neurol Neurosurg Psychiatry 1992;55:200–4.
25. Hahn RA. The nocebo phenomenon: concept, evidence, and implications for public health. Prev Med 1997;26:607–11.
26. Iverson GL, Lange RT, Brooks BL, et al. "Good old days" bias following mild traumatic brain injury. Clin Neuropsychol 2010;24:17–37.
27. Brooks BL, Kadoura B, Turley B, et al. Perception of recovery after pediatric mild traumatic brain injury is influenced by the "good old days" bias: tangible implications for clinical practice and outcomes research. Arch Clin Neuropsychol 2014; 29:186–93.
28. Babikian T, McArthur D, Asarnow RF. Predictors of 1-month and 1-year neurocognitive functioning from the UCLA longitudinal mild, uncomplicated, pediatric traumatic brain injury study. J Int Neuropsychol Soc 2013;19:145–54.
29. Bijur PE, Haslum M, Golding J. Cognitive outcomes of multiple mild head injuries in children. J Dev Behav Pediatr 1996;17:143–8.
30. Taylor HG, Dietrich A, Nuss K, et al. Post-concussive symptoms in children with mild traumatic brain injury. Neuropsychology 2010;24:148–59.
31. Testa JA, Malec JF, Moessner AM, et al. Predicting family functioning after TBI: impact of neurobehavioral factors. J Head Trauma Rehabil 2006;21:236–47.
32. Iverson GL, Zasler ND, Lange RT. Post-concussive disorder. In: Zasler ND, Katz DI, Zafonte RD, editors. Brain injury medicine: principles and practice. New York: Demos; 2007. p. 373–403.
33. Meares S, Shores EA, Taylor AJ, et al. The prospective course of postconcussion syndrome: the role of mild traumatic brain injury. Neuropsychology 2011;25:454.
34. Karr JE, Areshenkoff CN, Garcia-Barrera MA. The neuropsychological outcomes of concussion: a systematic review of meta-analyses on the cognitive sequelae of mild traumatic brain injury. Neuropsychology 2014;28:321.
35. Kirkwood MW, Peterson RL, Connery AK, et al. A pilot study investigating neuropsychological consultation as an intervention for persistent postconcussive symptoms in a pediatric sample. J Pediatr 2015. [Epub ahead of print].
36. Moor HM, Eisenhauer RC, Killian KD, et al. The relationship between adherence behaviors and recovery time in adolescents after a sports-related concussion: an observational study. Int J Sports Phys Ther 2015;10:225.
37. Thomas DG, Apps JN, Hoffmann RG, et al. Benefits of strict rest after acute concussion: a randomized controlled trial. Pediatrics 2015;135:213–23.
38. DiFazio M, Silverberg ND, Kirkwood MW, et al. Prolonged activity restriction after concussion are we worsening outcomes? Clin Pediatr 2015. [Epub ahead of print].
39. Bianchini KJ, Curtis KL, Greve KW. Compensation and malingering in traumatic brain injury: a dose-response relationship? Clin Neuropsychol 2006;20:831–47.
40. Green P, Rohling ML, Lees-Haley PR, et al. Effort has a greater effect on test scores than severe brain injury in compensation claimants. Brain Inj 2001;15: 1045–60.

41. Mittenberg W, Patton C, Canyock EM, et al. Base rates of malingering and symptom exaggeration. J Clin Exp Neuropsychol 2002;24:1094–102.

42. Kirkwood MW. A rationale for performance validity testing in child and adolescent assessment. In: Kirkwood MW, editor. Validity testing in child and adolescent assessment: evaluating exaggeration, feigning, and noncredible effort. New York: Guilford Publications; 2015. p. 3–21.

43. Kirkwood MW, Yeates KO, Randolph C, et al. The implications of symptom validity test failure for ability-based test performance in a pediatric sample. Psychol Assess 2012;24:36–45.

44. Kirkwood MW, Kirk JW. The base rate of suboptimal effort in a pediatric mild TBI sample: performance on the medical symptom validity test. Clin Neuropsychol 2010;24:860–72.

45. Binder LM, Rohling ML. Money matters: a meta-analytic review of the effects of financial incentives on recovery after closed-head injury. Am J Psychiatry 1996; 153:7–10.

46. Phillips T. The impact of litigation, regulation, and legislation on sport concussion management. Sport J; 2015. p. 8.

47. Alsalaheen B, Stockdale K, Pechumer D, et al. Measurement error in the Immediate Postconcussion Assessment and Cognitive Testing (ImPACT): systematic review. J Head Trauma Rehabil 2015. [Epub ahead of print].

48. Mayers LB, Redick TS. Clinical utility of ImPACT assessment for postconcussion return-to-play counseling: psychometric issues. J Clin Exp Neuropsychol 2012; 34:235–42.

49. Randolph C, McCrea M, Barr WB. Is neuropsychological testing useful in the management of sport-related concussion? J Athl Train 2005;40:139–52.

50. Randolph C. Baseline neuropsychological testing in managing sport-related concussion: does it modify risk? Curr Sports Med Rep 2011;10:21–6.

51. Barr WB. Neuropsychological testing of high school athletes: preliminary norms and test-retest indices. Arch Clin Neuropsychol 2003;18:91–101.

52. Broglio SP, Ferrara MS, Macciocchi SN, et al. Test-retest reliability of computerized concussion assessment programs. J Athl Train 2007;42:509–14.

53. Valovich McLeod TC, Bay RC, Heil J, et al. Identification of sport and recreational activity concussion history through the preparticipation screening and a symptom survey in young athletes. Clin J Sport Med 2008;18:235–40.

54. Bauer RM, Iverson GL, Cernich AN, et al. Computerized neuropsychological assessment devices: joint position paper of the American Academy of Clinical Neuropsychology and the National Academy of Neuropsychology. Clin Neuropsychol 2012;26:177–96.

55. Araujo GC, Antonini TN, Monahan K, et al. The relationship between suboptimal effort and post-concussion symptoms in children and adolescents with mild traumatic brain injury. Clin Neuropsychol 2014;28:786–801.

56. Larrabee GJ. Detection of malingering using atypical performance patterns on standard neuropsychological tests. Clin Neuropsychol 2003;17:410–25.

57. Kirkwood MW, Peterson RL, Connery AK, et al. Postconcussive symptom exaggeration after pediatric mild traumatic brain injury. Pediatrics 2014;133:643–50.

58. Lange RT, Iverson GL, Brooks BL, et al. Influence of poor effort on self-reported symptoms and neurocognitive test performance following mild traumatic brain injury. J Clin Exp Neuropsychol 2010;32:961–72.

59. Carone DA. Children with moderate/severe brain damage/dysfunction outperform adults with mild-to-no brain damage on the medical symptom validity test. Brain Inj 2008;22:960–71.

60. Donders J. Performance on the test of memory malingering in a mixed pediatric sample. Child Neuropsychol 2005;11:221–7.

61. Green P, Flaro L. Word memory test performance in children. Child Neuropsychol 2003;9:189–207.

62. Etherton JL, Bianchini KJ, Ciota MA, et al. Reliable digit span is unaffected by laboratory-induced pain: implications for clinical use. Assessment 2005;12:101–6.

63. Green P, Flaro L, Courtney J. Examining false positives on the word memory test in adults with mild traumatic brain injury. Brain Inj 2009;23:741–50.

64. Carone DA, Iverson GL, Bush SS. A model to approaching and providing feedback to patients regarding invalid test performance in clinical neuropsychological evaluations. Clin Neuropsychol 2010;24:759–78.

65. Connery A, Suchy Y. Managing noncredible performance in pediatric clinical assessment. In: Kirkwood MW, editor. Validity testing in child and adolescent assessment: evaluating exaggeration, feigning, and noncredible effort. New York: Guilford Publications; 2015. p. 145.

66. McCrea M, Iverson GL, McAllister TW, et al. An integrated review of recovery after mild traumatic brain injury (MTBI): implications for clinical management. Clin Neuropsychol 2009;23:1368–90.

67. McCrea M, Barr WB, Guskiewicz K, et al. Standard regression-based methods for measuring recovery after sport-related concussion. J Int Neuropsychol Soc 2005;11:58–69.

68. McCrea M, Kelly JP, Randolph C, et al. Standardized assessment of concussion (SAC): on-site mental status evaluation of the athlete. J Head Trauma Rehabil 1998;13:27–35.

69. Kirkwood MW, Yeates KO, Taylor HG, et al. Management of pediatric mild traumatic brain injury: a neuropsychological review from injury through recovery. Clin Neuropsychol 2008;22:769–800.

70. Dikmen S, Machamer J, Temkin N. Mild head injury: facts and artifacts. J Clin Exp Neuropsychol 2001;23:729–38.

71. Iverson GL, Lange RT. Examination of "postconcussion-like" symptoms in a healthy sample. Appl Neuropsychol 2003;10:137–44.

72. Kashluba S, Casey JE, Paniak C. Evaluating the utility of ICD-10 diagnostic criteria for postconcussion syndrome following mild traumatic brain injury. J Int Neuropsychol Soc 2006;12:111–8.

73. Lees-Haley PR, Fox DD, Courtney JC. A comparison of complaints by mild brain injury claimants and other claimants describing subjective experiences immediately following their injury. Arch Clin Neuropsychol 2001;16:689–95.

74. Gunstad J, Suhr JA. "Expectation as etiology" versus "the good old days": postconcussion syndrome symptom reporting in athletes, headache sufferers, and depressed individuals. J Int Neuropsychol Soc 2001;7:323–33.

75. Gouvier WD, Prestholdt PH, Warner MS. A survey of common misconceptions about head injury and recovery. Arch Clin Neuropsychol 1988;3:331–43.

76. Trahan DE, Ross CE, Trahan SL. Relationships among postconcussional-type symptoms, depression, and anxiety in neurologically normal young adults and victims of mild brain injury. Arch Clin Neuropsychol 2001;16:435–45.

77. Bryant RA. Posttraumatic stress disorder and mild brain injury: controversies, causes and consequences. J Clin Exp Neuropsychol 2001;23:718–28.

78. Hoge CW, McGurk D, Thomas JL, et al. Mild traumatic brain injury in US soldiers returning from Iraq. N Engl J Med 2008;358:453–63.

79. Landre N, Poppe CJ, Davis N, et al. Cognitive functioning and postconcussive symptoms in trauma patients with and without mild TBI. Arch Clin Neuropsychol 2006;21:255–73.

80. Moore EL, Terryberry-Spohr L, Hope DA. Mild traumatic brain injury and anxiety sequelae: a review of the literature. Brain Inj 2006;20:117–32.

81. Nicholson K, Martelli MF, Zasler ND. Does pain confound interpretation of neuropsychological test results? NeuroRehabilitation 2001;16:225–30.

82. O'Brien LM, Gozal D. Neurocognitive dysfunction and sleep in children: from human to rodent. Pediatr Clin North Am 2004;51:187–202.

83. Ponsford J. Rehabilitation interventions after mild head injury. Curr Opin Neurol 2005;18:692–7.

84. Ferguson RJ, Mittenberg W, Barone DF, et al. Postconcussion syndrome following sports-related head injury: expectation as etiology. Neuropsychology 1999;13: 582–9.

85. Mittenberg W, Canyock EM, Condit D, et al. Treatment of post-concussion syndrome following mild head injury. J Clin Exp Neuropsychol 2001;23:829–36.

86. Borg J, Holm L, Peloso PM, et al. Non-surgical intervention and cost for mild traumatic brain injury: results of the WHO Collaborating Centre Task Force on Mild Traumatic Brain Injury. J Rehabil Med Suppl 2004;36:76–83.

87. Comper P, Bisschop SM, Carnide N, et al. A systematic review of treatments for mild traumatic brain injury. Brain Inj 2005;19:863–80.

88. Bloom GA, Horton AS, McCrory P, et al. Sport psychology and concussion: new impacts to explore. Br J Sports Med 2004;38:519–21.

89. Dunn AL, Trivedi MH, O'Neal HA. Physical activity dose-response effects on outcomes of depression and anxiety. Med Sci Sports Exerc 2001;33(Suppl 6): S587–97 [discussion: 609–10].

90. Randolph C, Kirkwood MW. What are the real risks of sport-related concussion, and are they modifiable? J Int Neuropsychol Soc 2009;15:512–20.

91. Children's Hospital Colorado. Return to learn plan. 2014. Available at: http:// concussioncomeback.childrenscolorado.org. Accessed November 18, 2015.

Retirement and Activity Restrictions Following Concussion

Scott R. Laker, MD[a],*, Adele Meron, MD[a],
Michael R. Greher, PhD, ABPP-CN[b], Julie Wilson, MD[c]

KEYWORDS

- Concussion • Retirement • Activity restrictions • Sport-related concussion

KEY POINTS

- Return-to-play decisions in the setting of multiple concussions, prolonged recovery, or structural abnormalities should be individualized based on thorough history, imaging, medical workup, and specialist consultation.
- There are limited evidence-based guidelines to guide retirement decisions in the setting of athletes with multiple concussions or prolonged recoveries.
- There are consistent expert opinions regarding return to play in the setting of congenital and acquired structural abnormalities of the cervical spine and brain.
- Neuropsychological testing is a critical component in the workup of patients considering medical retirement.

INTRODUCTION

In recent years, concussion has been brought to the forefront of both public and scientific literature. This attention includes increased concern about removing athletes from the field of play following a concussion, along with establishment of return-to-play protocols for subsequent practices and competition.[1] In addition to these safeguards, which are thus far clinically rather than empirically driven, more players and physicians are being faced with the difficult question of how many concussions are too many to continue participation in a given sport. Now, in the wake of increased attention on the subject, players across several professional sports are electing to retire or terminate contracts because of concerns over the long-term consequences of concussion. As many athletes attempt to balance their passion for sport and financial security with their long-term health and safety, physicians are in the unique position to offer education and guidance around how many concussions are too many.

[a] Department of Physical Medicine and Rehabilitation, University of Colorado School of Medicine, Denver, CO 80045, USA; [b] University of Colorado School of Medicine, Department of Neurosurgery, Academic Office One, 12631 E. 17th Avenue, Suite 5001, Aurora, CO 80045, USA; [c] Children's Hospital Colorado, Aurora, CO, USA
* Corresponding author. Room 2513, Mail Stop F493, Denver, CO 80045.
E-mail address: scott.laker@ucdenver.edu

Phys Med Rehabil Clin N Am 27 (2016) 487–501
http://dx.doi.org/10.1016/j.pmr.2016.01.001
1047-9651/16/$ – see front matter © 2016 Elsevier Inc. All rights reserved.

pmr.theclinics.com

EPIDEMIOLOGY

The Centers for Disease Control and Prevention estimates that there are between 1.6 and 3.8 million recreation and sport-related concussions per year.[2] Marar and colleagues[3] studied high school athletes over a 2-year period and found concussions occurred at a rate of 2.5 per 10,000 athlete exposures. Football had both the highest number of concussions (47%) and the highest rate of concussion (6.4 per 10,000 exposures). The sport with the greatest proportion of concussions compared with other injuries was boys' ice hockey (22%). In sex-comparable sports, girls had a higher concussion rate (1.7) than boys (1.0). Overall, 11.5% of athletes sustaining a concussion had previously sustained a sports-related concussion in either that season or a previous season. Most athletes (55.3%) returned to play in 1 to 3 weeks, with 22.8% returning in less than 1 week and 2.0% returning in less than 1 day.[3] In a 2014 survey of Division I National Collegiate Athletic Association athletes, 11.7% reported one concussion and 4.5% reported multiple concussions during their collegiate career. The highest rates were in women's and men's ice hockey, wrestling, and football. The highest reported rate of multiple concussions was in football.[4]

In professional sports, the stakes and financial incentives are higher. There were 228 reported concussions in the 2013 National Football League season, including preseason and regular season games and practices.[5] The National Hockey League (NHL) saw 559 concussions from the 1997 through 2004 seasons totaling 1.8 concussions per 1000 player hours.[6] There were 53 concussions in the 2014 NHL season, down from 78 in the previous season.[7]

PAST AND CURRENT RECOMMENDATIONS

The question of when to retire following sport-related concussion is not a new one. Historically, recommendations were based on a proposal by Quigley in 1945, which was later published by Thorndike[8] in 1952. This article suggested that play should be suspended for at least the remainder of the season if an athlete sustained 3 concussions. At the time, concussion required a loss of consciousness. Although these recommendations were based on anecdotal evidence and using a concussion definition that we no longer consider valid, they have been used as the basis for current return-to-play guidelines, league protocols, medical decision making, as well as the hypothetical threshold for research into the cumulative effects of repeated injury. In 2002, McCrory[9] published a review questioning the scientific validity of the 3-strike rule and suggesting that there is no set number of concussions after which a player should retire. A general set of guidelines was proposed based on common clinical scenarios, including the recommendations that players with persistent cognitive or neurologic symptoms should be withheld from collision sports until symptoms fully resolve and also highlighting the importance of differentiating postconcussive headaches from headaches with an alternative cause.

McCrory[9] proposed that moderate to severe traumatic brain injury (TBI) resulting in subarachnoid hemorrhage (SAH), persistent neurologic deficit, or TBI requiring craniotomy should be a contraindication to further participation in collision sport. Recommendations for moderate TBI resulting in epidural hematoma include reevaluation for participation in collision sport after a minimum of 12 months. If symptoms have resolved and neurologic sequelae have normalized, return to play may be considered.[9]

Cantu and Register-Mihalik[10] published a statement in 2011 addressing the issue of retirement from sport following concussion. Contraindications to returning to sports were persistent postconcussive symptoms, increasing symptoms in the setting of decreasing impacts, symptomatic neurologic or pain-producing abnormalities about the foramen magnum, permanent central neurologic sequelae, hydrocephalus, spontaneous SAH from any cause, and second impact syndrome (SIS).[10] Of note, the topic of SIS remains both controversial and questionable, as evidence for such a phenomenon is minimal based on critical review of these cases.[11–13] These observations raise critical questions about the validity of SIS as a criterion for retirement from sport.

In 2011, Sedney and colleagues[14] published a review of the current literature and offered a list of specific season-ending and career-ending features of concussion. Season-ending features included prolonged postconcussion syndrome (PCS) (defined as symptoms >6 months, lowered concussion threshold, diminished athletic or academic performance), 3 or more concussions or 2 or more major concussions (symptomatic for longer than a week) in a single season, or diminished academic or athletic performance. Career-ending features included persistent PCS (without a clear definition of persistence), Chiari malformation, intracranial hemorrhage, diminished academic performance or cognitive abilities, lowered threshold for concussion, 3 or more major concussions, computed tomography or MRI evidence of structural abnormality, nonresolving MRI deficits, or symptoms of chronic traumatic encephalopathy (CTE). The investigators emphasized the potential for cumulative and, rarely, progressive symptoms after concussion.[14]

Concannon and colleagues[15] reviewed the subject in 2014, creating a similar list of absolute contraindications to return to play, including persistent PCS (with PCS defined as symptoms lasting longer than 3 months), SAH, permanent neurologic injury, SIS, hydrocephalus, imaging that increases risk for future brain injury (edema, hemorrhage, hydrocephalus, arachnoid cysts), and permanent deficit on neuropsychological testing. On the topic of in vivo diagnosis of CTE as a criterion for return to play, this article called into question the actual incidence and prevalence of CTE, emphasizing the clinical variability in symptoms and weak correlation between symptoms and histopathology of tissue samples.[15] The investigators recommended further study into risk factors for developing CTE as well as the actual incidence and prevalence. These same questions and other critical issues have been raised with regard to CTE, which thus far remain unanswered.[16–19] Given the preliminary nature of the evidence, it remains premature to use CTE (or symptoms presumed to be related to this condition) as a criterion for clinical decision making, including retirement from a given sport. The investigators do recommend discussing the current state of this diagnosis with families as the literature base evolves.

Although some of the recommendations for retirement from sport have a strong evidence base and others are consistent among experts, such as SAH, some of the cited recommendations need clarification. Persistent neurologic deficits and persistent symptoms provide a vague timeline, which cannot easily be enforced when a player is exhibiting a prolonged recovery. Although it is clear that a player should not return to play while symptomatic, a prolonged recovery in itself does not necessitate retirement. It is not clear at what point in time symptoms or deficits become persistent and, thus, become a contraindication to return to play. Additionally, although in the past Chiari malformations were thought to preclude athletes from participating in collision sport, recent studies have shown that small asymptomatic Chiari malformations provide no additional neurologic risk to collision sport athletes.[20] There is some question in regard to the return to play in the setting of craniotomy. Multiple reports of safe return to play in multiple sports exist.[21]

PROLONGED SYMPTOMS

PCS is a feared yet poorly understood consequence of concussion in sport. Of those who sustain concussions, 95% or more resolve within a few days to around a 3-month time period, leaving a small minority (5% or less) of concussed athletes with prolonged symptoms. Who of these will be diagnosed with PCS is uncertain because of inconsistencies in definition and the contribution of confounding diagnoses. A recent survey of American College of Sports Medicine physicians highlighted the lack of consensus over the duration and quantity of symptoms required to make the diagnosis of PCS. The greatest proportion of physicians surveyed (33%) replied that they make the diagnosis after 1 to 3 months of symptoms; however, 27% selected "less than 2 weeks" and 20% selected the "2 weeks to 1 month" option.[22] This lack of consensus carries over into retirement recommendations that use prolonged symptoms as a criterion for retirement. Several sources cite persistent symptoms as a condition for retirement; however, few quantify how many weeks or months of symptoms qualify as persistent. Care must also be taken in making this diagnosis, as there are many conditions that could be falsely designated as sequelae of concussion. Preexisting headache and mood disorders can be misattributed to the concussive injury and obscure the trajectory of the recovery, leading to incorrect diagnoses, failure to treat these conditions, and misguided recommendations to athletes regarding return to play and retirement.

Iverson calculated the effect size of a wide variety of nonconcussive-related factors across several meta-analyses (eg, chronic benzodiazepine use/withdrawal; psychiatric conditions, such as bipolar disorder, attention-deficit/hyperactivity disorder [ADHD], and depression; and litigation). These factors had substantially greater impact on neuropsychological functioning than concussion following the 3-month recovery window. Nonathlete studies have demonstrated that preexisting psychiatric illness or mood disorder as well as high anxiety levels 1 week after injury both correlated with unresolved symptoms at 3 months.[23] There are few factors that may be predictive of prolonged recovery including symptom score at presentation,[24] age,[25] amnesia,[25] photophobia, phonophobia, and history of migraines.[26] Although it would be clinically useful to be able to predict the onset of a prolonged recovery, there are more questions to be answered in order to make evidence-based retirement recommendations based on prolonged recovery in athletes.

The questions that continue to elude us are as follows: Is there increased risk associated with having symptoms that persist outside of the normal recovery period and do these risks resolve once the symptoms have resolved? These answers likely lie in the physiologic mechanism of recovery. We know there is a window of metabolic vulnerability following concussion whereby the brain experiences a high cerebral energy state with altered glucose metabolism, cerebral perfusion, and cellular hypofunction.[27] We do not yet know whether these metabolic changes are altered in prolonged recovery and, if so, what vulnerability is imparted and for what duration or if persistent symptoms are entirely unrelated to such metabolic changes much as the neuropsychological literature suggests the importance of non-neurological factors.

There is no evidence to suggest that a player who experiences prolonged symptoms after a concussion will have an abnormal recovery following subsequent concussions. So what is the real risk to returning an athlete to play after their symptoms have resolved? Many successful athletes have missed months of play and returned to their sport without further apparent consequence. Based on the current evidence, the authors recommend that players with prolonged recovery (persistence of symptoms outside the typical 10-day recovery) are worked up for other causes of their symptoms and not returned to play until concussion-related symptoms have resolved.

CUMULATIVE EFFECTS OF CONCUSSION

Although there is significant evidence that athletes who have sustained concussions are at increased risk for future concussions and mildly slower recovery of symptoms,[28] the evidence for cumulative effects of multiple concussions is less conclusive. The possibility exists that there are no cumulative effects of repeat concussion and that, once a concussion has healed, the metabolic activity in the brain is reset to baseline. However, there are also differing yet not mutually exclusive theories that describe static and progressive neurologic changes following repeat concussion. The breadth of research on the subject is growing, but we have yet to reach a consensus on the effect of multiple injuries to an athlete's brain.

Several studies have examined the effects of multiple concussions on symptom presentation at subsequent concussion. Collins and colleagues[29] reported in 2002 that athletes with 3 or more prior concussions (self-reported via standardized concussion history form) were more likely to experience on-field loss of consciousness (LOC), anterograde amnesia, and confusion following a concussion and were 9.3 times more likely to have 3 to 4 symptoms following subsequent concussion than those athletes with fewer concussions.[29] Brooks and colleagues[30] studied the effects of multiple concussions on adolescent athletes and found that, among athletes 13 to 17 years old, there were significantly more reported baseline symptoms, however, no significant difference on neurocognitive testing in athletes with 2 or more reported prior concussions. Guskiewicz and colleagues[28] performed a large-scale study of 2905 college football players over 3 seasons and identified 196 concussions in 184 athletes. This study showed evidence for susceptibility to repeat concussion within the typical concussion recovery period. Eleven of 12 (92%) repeat concussions occurred within 10 days of the initial injury. Statistical analysis revealed that athletes with 3 or more prior concussions (by self-report) were 3 times more likely to sustain a concussion than those with no concussion history. This study also measured duration of symptoms and found that athletes with prior concussions experienced slightly longer recovery than those with no concussions (greater than 1 week more).[28]

In a study of high school athletes, grouped by number of prior concussions, it was shown that those with a history of 2 or more concussions had higher rates of headaches, balance problems, and dizziness than players with 1 or no concussions. They also reported higher rates of physical symptoms and symptoms associated with sleep. Those with a history of 2 or more concussions reported higher ratings on nausea and fatigue compared with those with no history of concussion.[31] However, the studies mentioned earlier used self-report as a means to determine incidence of prior concussion, which inherently diminishes the validity of their outcomes. Furthermore, several studies conducted to date do not reflect a relationship between previous mild TBIs (MTBIs) and persistent PCS symptoms.[32–35] It is also well understood that the symptoms of PCS are nonspecific and, therefore, highly problematic for the purpose of clinical diagnosis as well as in conducting research on outcomes from concussion. A strong body of literature from sport and nonsport literature has developed that shows high rates of postconcussive symptoms in association with non-neurological factors, such as orthopedic injuries, psychological problems (eg, posttraumatic stress disorder and depression), involvement in personal injury claims, and even healthy controls.[36–41] Given these complexities, consultation with a neuropsychologist is oftentimes quite helpful to assist with the differential diagnosis of concussion based on acute symptoms at the time of injury and to objectively assess cognitive functions rather than rely on self-reported symptoms to determine the effects of injury and best course of treatment moving forward. Additional benefits of such consultations are described further later.

Although no animal brain can serve as a perfect model for humans, animal models allow us to examine pathophysiologic correlations under conditions we are unable to reproduce in human models. One animal model attempted to characterize the effects of cumulative head trauma in mice and demonstrated that repeated mild closed head injury (mCHI) in mice worsened vestibulomotor, motor, short-term memory, and conflict learning impairments as compared with a single mCHI. These learning and memory impairments were sustained 3 months after injury. In this study, repeated mCHIs also reduced cerebral perfusion, prolonged the inflammatory response, and, in some animals, caused hippocampal neuronal loss.[42]

Luo and colleagues[43] demonstrated that animals that received repetitive MTBI showed a significant impairment in spatial learning and memory when tested at 2 and 6 months after injury. Astrogliosis and increased p-Tau immunoreactivity were observed on postmortem pathologic examinations in mice that sustained 3 impacts versus sham mice. Astrogliosis increased with increasing number of MTBIs.[43]

In a series of animal and human studies, Vagnozzi and colleagues[44] have shown the value of magnetic resonance spectroscopy in evaluating the metabolic changes within the brain following multiple concussive injuries with variable spacing. These studies demonstrated that the metabolic effect of recurrent concussion was maximized with a 3-day separation in rats. Although animal models continue to provide insight into the pathologic effects of cumulative brain injury, there has yet to be a study to evaluate the influence of time between concussions on recovery time to account for the effect of healing following the primary concussion.[44]

Neuropsychological Testing

The evidence to date on persistent cognitive deficits as a function of multiple MTBI events is equivocal. A meta-analysis of 8 studies on the cumulative effects of concussion in athletes, involving 614 cases of multiple MTBIs and 926 control cases of a single MTBI, demonstrated that the overall effect of multiple MTBIs on neuropsychological functioning was minimal. Follow-up analyses revealed an association between multiple self-reported MTBIs and lower scores in executive functions and delayed memory, but the investigators also noted that the effect sizes were small and results were of unclear clinical relevance.[45] Iverson and colleagues[46] compared athletes with 3 or more concussions with those with fewer concussions, all of whom completed testing in 4 domains of neurocognitive functioning during a preseason baseline. Analysis revealed that working memory was significantly different between the two groups, but the investigators noted several critical methodological limitations and themselves described the findings as nonpursuasive.[46] In addition, several studies have found that a history of multiple MTBIs was not associated with greater difficulty on neuropsychological testing. For example, Bruce and Echemendia[32] grouped 479 male collegiate athletes into those with 1, 2, or more than 2 concussions, with no impact on traditional neuropsychological measures of memory, processing speed, mental flexibility, and executive functioning.[32] Similarly, Iverson and colleagues[35] conducted computerized neurocognitive testing with 867 high school and college male athletes and found no significant differences in performance between those with 1 or 2 concussions. A similar finding was recently discovered in children aged 8 to 16 years, including those with 1, 2, or 3 or more previous concussions.[47] In light of these fairly discrepant findings, it remains unclear whether a threshold exists after which repeated MTBIs results in persistent cognitive deficits. If so, the literature to date suggests that the effects are likely small and may be specific to a certain subset of the population, which has thus far not been identified.[47,48] Perhaps most important, the authors are unaware of any prospective studies investigating differential neuropsychological outcomes for individuals who have retired from a given sport because of multiple MTBI histories at one time point or another in the course of these injuries.

Given the absence of any clear evidence basis for application with patients, practitioners are left to make recommendations regarding retirement from a sport based on sound clinical judgment. This judgment should likely be based on consideration of multiple factors similar to several suggestions already highlighted earlier, including the number of known concussions, severity of the injuries, and the presence of increasingly prolonged recovery from symptoms with successive MTBI events. Kirkwood and colleagues[19] offer a list of questions to address when considering disqualification of an athlete. This list includes the following:

> *1. Are concussions occurring closer together in time? 2. Are concussions occurring as a result of a lesser blow or impact (eg, the impact that caused the most recent concussion would not have caused an injury 3 years ago)? 3. Is the rate of recovery slower after each concussion? 4. Is there incomplete recovery after a concussion (eg, only getting back to 80% of typical functioning)? 5. Is there a persisting decline in academic, cognitive, social, emotional, or other personal function after a concussion?[19]*

With regard to neuropsychological testing in particular, the potential benefits of these examinations include offering the opportunity to objectively track cognitive status over the course of repeated injuries to determine the cognitive impact of these events. Neuropsychological examination is also likely to be helpful in identifying alternative factors that could account for persistent cognitive complaints beyond the typical recovery window or worsening complaints. Such factors include preexisting or postinjury psychological challenges as well as performance and symptom validity issues that sometimes arise.[19] As in cases involving questions about timing of return to play, the topic of baseline cognitive testing seems reasonable to address in the context of retirement from a sport due to repeated concussion. Several methodological concerns remain about the use of baseline testing, and the data are currently lacking with regard to any indications of improved outcomes as a function of use of baseline testing.[49,50] Nevertheless, such testing may be valuable in select cases for the purpose of aiding in detecting a clear downward trajectory over repeated injuries and associated serial testing sessions in which alternate/non-neurological explanations do not seem to account for these changes. However, it is also critical to recognize the significant psychometric limitations of many of the current computerized measures available today in particular (as compared with more traditional neuropsychological tests) and the lack of scientific data to suggest that such measures modify the risk on return to play.[49,50] Despite the remaining questions about the scientific validity of baseline computerized testing, it has become fairly commonplace in a variety of collegiate and professional sports settings.

Clearly, a conservative approach is the most recommendable course of action in making decisions about retirement from a given sport. As applied in neuropsychological testing in particular, unequivocal evidence of worsening cognitive outcomes over the course of repeated injuries and serial examinations conducted at similar time points during recovery from each respective event is certainly a reasonable basis for recommending retirement from a given sport; this could include increasingly longer periods of cognitive deficit or worsening cognitive decline on neuropsychological testing after each successive injury.

MODIFYING FACTORS

Medical conditions, including migraines, ADHD, learning disabilities, sleep disorders, and depression and other mental health disorders, are factors that may impact an athlete's recovery from concussion.[1,51] These conditions have not definitively been shown to increase an athlete's risk for sustaining a concussion but may contribute to ongoing symptoms after an injury. To date, it is unclear if these conditions themselves are responsible for an increased symptom severity profile or if athletes with these conditions experience a more complicated concussion course.[51,52] Poor control of coexisting medical conditions before injury may complicate recovery. Clinicians caring for these athletes should be aware that many will not be entirely asymptomatic on recovery; however, return to baseline status is necessary before considering return to sports.[10] Currently, there are no guidelines discussing how these conditions factor into a retirement decision; rather, the overall impact of multiple concussions and coexisting medical conditions on each individual athlete should be considered.

Female sex is associated with an increased risk of concussion in certain sports[3,52]; but the literature is mixed regarding its relationship with prolonged symptoms or cognitive recovery,[10,53] so sex is not clearly a factor in retirement decisions. However, an athlete's age may impact return to play decisions and is discussed in further detail later.

PEDIATRIC ATHLETES

Young athletes deserve special consideration related to several factors, including ongoing brain development and changing cognitive function, variability in symptom reporting, and reliance on adults to access medical care.[1,10,51,53,54] Furthermore, many young athletes participate in more than one sport, although there is an increasing trend toward early sport specialization, both of which may complicate a return-to-sport decision.[55] In addition, young athletes may have a higher number of future athletic exposures relative to college or professional athletes.[10] Therefore, experts typically recommend a more conservative return-to-play plan when returning young athletes to physical activity; but specific guidelines are currently lacking in the literature.[1,53,56] Factors such as the timing, duration, and severity of concussions as well as the patient-specific modifiers listed earlier should be considered.

Younger age has been associated with longer duration of cognitive recovery from concussion, even with the first injury.[56] A review of the pediatric literature by Kirkwood and colleagues[19] suggests some data indicate a slightly slower recovery for high school athletes compared with adults (by a magnitude of a few days), whereas others suggest similar outcomes between these groups. Eisenberg and colleagues[57] demonstrated that timing of injury affects concussion recovery, reporting an increased duration of symptoms for patients aged 11 to 22 years with a history of previous concussion in the last year. Neuroimaging with MRI may be considered for patients with persistent symptoms, as this may reveal a structural injury that could have implications regarding safe return to full athletic activity.[58] The assistance of a pediatric neuropsychologist with expertise in concussion evaluation in documenting the presence or absence of neurocognitive deficits is invaluable in retirement decisions.

Sport-related concussions and persistent postconcussion symptoms up to 12 months after injury negatively impact the quality of life in children and adolescents, although the reasons for such a protracted period of recovery are unlikely to be the direct result of a single concussion and other complicating factors should always be explored.[59,60] Furthermore, many young athletes derive a strong sense of self from participation in sports; hence, retirement or disqualification from athletic activity should be decided after carefully considering the history and potential complicating factors and weighing risks and benefits. DiFazio and colleagues[61] discuss the potential harms of prolonged rest in the setting of concussion treatment, including an increased risk for depression resulting from prolonged activity restriction. Therefore, return to low-risk physical activity should still be encouraged even if an athlete is not able to return to competitive sports.

When the decision is made for a young athlete to be temporarily or permanently disqualified from a competitive sport, effort should be made to maintain peer relationships and social engagement, with careful attention for evolution of mental health concerns. In certain cases, consideration may be given to changing competition level (club to recreational), decreasing from year-round to single-season participation, or changing positions (catcher to outfield) as a means to modify risk of future injury.[62]

Future athletic exposures also factor into return-to-play decisions. For example, a high school volleyball athlete with a history of 3 previous concussions over 5 years may be allowed to complete his or her senior season, whereas a middle school football athlete with his or her second concussion of the season is advised to delay return to contact sports until the next competitive season in order to limit exposure for additional injury. Furthermore, patients should be counseled regarding the potential for concussion outside of sport-related activity, as injuries may occur on the playground, in physical education classes, and during recreational activity, such as snow sports, skateboarding, and riding a bicycle.

DISCUSSION

Retirement from sport or retirement from collision/contact sports is often an important and challenging decision for athletes and their families to consider. Providers have limited guidance when advising patients in these scenarios. We must ask ourselves why we are recommending retirement. Are we concerned for permanent cognitive deficit, prolonged future recoveries, increasingly severe symptoms during the next concussion, permanent injury/symptoms, or an ultimate diagnosis of CTE? In many cases, the issue may be a lack of experience with what are rare scenarios. Each of these potential situations must be weighed by the provider and discussed with patients. However, do these situations warrant absolute contraindications, relative contraindications, or no contraindication? For example, a youth athlete with a strong family history of hypertrophic cardiomyopathy may not be medically allowed to participate in sports regardless of the wishes of the family. The well-documented incidence of sudden cardiac death outweighs the potential benefits of participating in certain sports. Concussions are clearly different, and the risks of long-term (and even shorter-term) consequences of sports related concussion (SRC) are not as well understood.

The authors do not recommend any return to play in the setting of athletes who have ongoing symptoms attributed to the concussion itself. The authors propose that athletes who continue to note symptoms be worked up for all other potential causes using MRI, blood work, neuropsychological screening, and often times referral for thorough specialist evaluation (**Box 1**).

Although some studies have demonstrated sex-related differences in concussion risk, the authors recommend that the sex of the athlete should not play a role in retirement decisions. The authors do recommend altering retirement recommendations based on age, as the young athlete brain is still developing and younger athletes have more potential future exposures. The authors strongly recommend neuropsychological testing as part of a young athlete's return-to-play decision in cases in which

---

Box 1
Workup in cases in which medical retirement is considered (eg, multiple concussions, prolonged recovery, multiple modifying factors, concern or direct findings of structural abnormalities)

Initial workup for potential medical retirement

- MRI brain
- Formal neuropsychological examination with consultation and recommendations
- Medical workup including common mimics of PCS (eg, basic blood work screening, including complete blood count, comprehensive metabolic panel (CMP), thyroid function, and so forth)

Secondary workup for potential medical retirement

- MRI cervical spine as indicated
- Further medical workup as indicated
- Specialist consultation as indicated (eg, sports medicine, neurosurgery, psychology, psychiatry, and so forth)

---

retirement is considered. If retirement is recommended for a young athlete, there should be social interventions to prevent the isolation that can occur from loss of the team environment. To prevent the onset of mood disorders as a result of physical inactivity, the authors promote continued low-risk exercise.

The published retirement guidelines are thoughtful and considerate, though are limited to expert opinion. In many cases, there will likely be no controlled studies that will guide these decisions in the future (ie, studies on craniotomy, return to play after >5 concussions, and so forth). The strongest recommendations are in regard to significant intracranial pathology (eg, subdural hematoma, SAH) and congenital anomalies of the foramen magnum in which consequences may be catastrophic (see **Box 1**). The authors suggest that, in many of these situations, retirement should be recommended to patients and families. However, we must clearly recognize the limitations of the evidence base when discussing the finality of retirement from sport, especially given the level of play.

The clinical differences between an athlete with an SAH and another with persistent symptoms secondary to uncomplicated concussion are vast, though the published recommendation to retire would be the same. As discussed throughout the article, the concept of *persistent symptoms* following concussion varies widely throughout published literature and across physician practice. We must have some perspective on these situations lest we prematurely retire youth and young adult athletes from sports that have a multitude of clearly defined positive effects because of concern of poorly defined, albeit possible, negative outcomes.

Athletes with multiple concussions are the most common scenarios in which retirement will be discussed. Current retirement recommendations regarding the number of concussions are based on studies that suggest prolonged recoveries and worsened sideline presentation combined with common sense concepts about the consequences of multiple brain injuries. Although these concerns are real and important, we struggle with understanding the consequences of multiple concussions. There are developing data that are concerning for the long-term consequences of concussions and even subconcussive blows. However, the authors would argue that it is premature to make retirement decisions solely based on the incomplete, current literature base with regard to multiple concussions. Each athlete who presents with multiple concussions must be treated individually, including past medical history, modifying factors, future goals and career plans, and their history of concussions. The authors recommend that these athletes be worked up thoroughly for early signs that could suggest more prolonged issues (**Box 2**). Currently, the authors consider 3 to 4 concussions the bellwether to begin discussions for retirement from contact and collision sport and potentially changing to a less concussion-prone sport. It is the authors' experience that one episode of prolonged recovery may have no bearing on the recovery of subsequent concussions. However, in the setting of multiple concussions with consistently prolonged recovery and decreased injury threshold, the authors do suggest moving to less risky sports or full retirement for collision and contact sports. Based on the current state of the science, the authors' concern is focused more on the direct impact of prolonged recovery on the rest of their academic, social, and work life rather than the potential for permanent, long-term consequence.

The authors' preferred framework is to discuss the best available evidence applicable to the individual athlete (eg, professional data for professional athletes, collegiate data for collegiate athletes, and youth data for youth athletes). The authors discuss the current understanding of cognitive and somatic complaints in similar situations, whether that is prolonged recoveries, multiple concussions, multiple modifying factors, or structural abnormalities. The athlete is given the potential outcomes of return to play, both clear and unclear (eg, including clear risks of increased concussion rates in athletes with multiple concussions vs the far less clear potential concerns for permanent neurologic disease). The authors routinely use formal neuropsychological professionals and subspecialist consultation when needed to guide these decisions.

The authors reserve formal medical retirement (ie, athlete may not return to play regardless of athlete's desire to do so) for athletes with structural abnormalities that imply potentially catastrophic outcomes with collision sport (not necessarily only related to TBI), athletes with persistent or worsening abnormalities on objective pen and paper neuropsychological examination following repeated events, and athletes with persistent neurologic sequelae. Currently, the authors recommend that the decision to return to play in the setting of craniotomy be individualized based on the level of play (ie, professional athletes should be considered differently than amateur and youth athletes) and input from the neurosurgical and sports medicine team, though erring on the side of caution should be considered the norm. The authors have proposed a framework for retirement considerations, though this should be highly individualized and is not meant to be solely algorithmic (**Fig. 1**). Discussion of permanent and

---

Box 2
List of conditions and scenarios in which medical retirement should be strongly considered or recommended

- SAH
- Unresolved subdural hematoma
- Unresolved epidural hematoma
- Craniotomy[a]
- Symptomatic Chiari malformation
- Permanent neurologic sequelae
- Persistent or worsening deficits on formal neuropsychological examination over the course of repeated injuries, concluded to be secondary to neurologic injury

[a] Craniotomy patients have been known to return to play without issue, though data are limited. Recommend neurosurgical consultation in all of these cases.

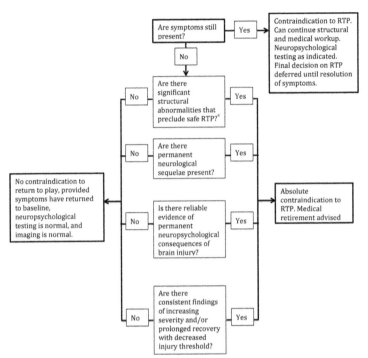

Fig. 1. Proposed retirement consideration algorithm. MRI, neuropsychological testing, and medical workup for other potential causes of symptoms are part of this workup. [a] Including (but not limited to) SAH, pain-producing abnormalities in the foramen magnum, hydrocephalus, and prior craniotomy for subdural hematoma. RTP, return to play.

potentially life-threatening consequences should be a clear and well-documented part of patient instruction. In many cases, the authors formally recommend obtaining multiple opinions.

REFERENCES

1. McCrory P, Meeuwisse WH, Aubry M, et al. Consensus statement on concussion in sport: the 4th International Conference on Concussion in Sport held in Zurich, November 2012. Br J Sports Med 2013;47(5):250–8.
2. Faul M, Xu L, Wald M, et al. Traumatic brain injury in the United States: emergency department visits, hospitalizations and deaths 2002–2006. U S Dep Heal Hum Serv ices Centers D isease Control Prev ion. 2010. Available at: http://www.cdc.gov/traumaticbraininjury/pdf/blue_book.pdf. Accessed September 16, 2015.
3. Marar M, McIlvain NM, Fields SK, et al. Epidemiology of concussions among United States high school athletes in 20 sports. Am J Sports Med 2012;40(4):747–55.
4. Bell L, Hwang S, Paskus T. Self-reported concussion among NCAA student-athletes executive summary February 2014. 2014:3–5. Available at: https://www.ncaa.org/sites/default/files/Concussion GOALS Exec Summary_Feb_12_2014_FINALpost_0.pdf. Accessed November 9, 2015.
5. Garriott K. NFL says concussions, ACL injuries decreased this season. NFL.com. 2014. Available at: http://www.nfl.com/news/story/0ap2000000320373/article/nfl-says-concussions-acl-injuries-decreased-this-season. Accessed September 16, 2015.

6. Benson BW, Meeuwisse WH, Rizos J, et al. A prospective study of concussions among National Hockey League players during regular season games: the NHL-NHLPA concussion program. CMAJ 2011;183(8):905–11.

7. Wisniewski J. NHL still grappling with concussions. Assoc Press; 2014. Available at: http://espn.go.com/nhl/playoffs/2014/story/_/id/11051889/nhl-says-concussions-decreased-protocol-remains-imperfect. Accessed September 1, 2015.

8. Thorndike A. Serious recurrent injuries of athletes. N Engl J Med 1952;247(15): 554–6.

9. McCrory P. 2002 Refshauge lecture. When to retire after concussion? J Sci Med Sport 2002;5(3):169–82.

10. Cantu RC, Register-Mihalik JK. Considerations for return-to-play and retirement decisions after concussion. PM R 2011;3(10 Suppl 2):S440–4.

11. Mccrory PR, Berkovic SF. Second impact syndrome. Neurology 1998;50(3): 677–83.

12. McCrory P, Davis G, Makdissi M. Second impact syndrome or cerebral swelling after sporting head injury. Curr Sports Med Rep 2012;11(1):21–3.

13. Kirkwood MW, Randolph C, Yeates KO. Sport-related concussion: a call for evidence and perspective amidst the alarms. Clin J Sport Med 2012;22(5):383–4.

14. Sedney CL, Orphanos J, Bailes JE. When to consider retiring an athlete after sports-related concussion. Clin Sports Med 2011;30(1):189–200.

15. Concannon LG, Kaufman MS, Herring SA. The million dollar question: when should an athlete retire after concussion? Curr Sports Med Rep 2014;13(6): 365–9.

16. Randolph C. Is chronic traumatic encephalopathy a real disease? Curr Sports Med Rep 2014;13(1):33–7.

17. Davis GA, Castellani RJ, McCrory P. Neurodegeneration and sport. Neurosurgery 2015;76(6):643–6.

18. Wortzel HS, Brenner LA, Arciniegas DB. Traumatic brain injury and chronic traumatic encephalopathy: a forensic neuropsychiatric perspective. Behav Sci Law 2013;31(6):721–38.

19. Kirkwood MW, Randolph C, McCrea M, et al. Sport-related concussion. In: Kirkwood MW, Yeates KO, editors. Mild traumatic brain injury in children and adolescents: from basic science to clinical management. New York: Guilford Press; 2012. p. 341–60.

20. Meehan WP, Jordaan M, Prabhu SP, et al. Risk of athletes with Chiari malformations suffering catastrophic injuries during sports participation is low. Clin J Sport Med 2014;25(2):133–7.

21. Miele VJ, Bailes JE, Martin NA. Participation in contact or collision sports in athletes with epilepsy, genetic risk factors, structural brain lesions, or history of craniotomy. Neurosurg Focus 2006;21(4):1–8.

22. Rose SC, Fischer AN, Heyer GL. How long is too long? The lack of consensus regarding the post-concussion syndrome diagnosis. Brain Inj 2015;29(7–8): 798–803.

23. Ponsford J, Cameron P, Fitzgerald M, et al. Predictors of postconcussive symptoms 3 months after mild traumatic brain injury. Neuropsychology 2012;26(3): 304–13.

24. Meehan WP, Mannix RC, Stracciolini A, et al. Symptom severity predicts prolonged recovery after sport-related concussion, but age and amnesia do not. J Pediatr 2013;163(3):721–5.

25. Field M, Collins MW, Lovell MR, et al. Does age play a role in recovery from sports-related concussion? A comparison of high school and collegiate athletes. J Pediatr 2003;142(5):546–53.
26. Chrisman SP, Rivara FP, Schiff MA, et al. Risk factors for concussive symptoms 1 week or longer in high school athletes. Brain Inj 2013;27(1):1–9.
27. Barkhoudarian G, Hovda DA, Giza CC. The molecular pathophysiology of concussive brain injury. Clin Sports Med 2011;30(1):33–48.
28. Guskiewicz K, Mccrea M, Marshall SW, et al. Cumulative effects associated with recurrent concussion in collegiate football players: the NCAA concussion study. J Am Med Assoc 2003;290(19):2549–55.
29. Collins MW, Lovell MR, Iverson GL, et al. Cumulative effects of concussion in high school athletes. Neurosurgery 2002;51(5):1175–9.
30. Brooks BL, McKay CD, Mrazik M, et al. Subjective, but not objective, lingering effects of multiple past concussions in adolescents. J Neurotrauma 2013; 30(17):1469–75.
31. Schatz P, Moser RS, Covassin T, et al. Early indicators of enduring symptoms in high school athletes with multiple previous concussions. Neurosurgery 2011; 68(6):1562–7 [discussion: 1567].
32. Bruce JM, Echemendia RJ. History of multiple self-reported concussions is not associated with reduced cognitive abilities. Neurosurgery 2009;64(1):100–6 [discussion: 106].
33. Macciocchi SN, Barth JT, Littlefield L, et al. Multiple concussions and neuropsychological functioning in collegiate football players. J Athl Train 2001;36(3): 303–6.
34. McCrea M, Guskiewicz K, Randolph C, et al. Incidence, clinical course, and predictors of prolonged recovery time following sport-related concussion in high school and college athletes. J Int Neuropsychol Soc 2013;19(1):22–33.
35. Iverson GL, Brooks BL, Collins MW, et al. Tracking neuropsychological recovery following concussion in sport. Brain Inj 2006;20(3):245–52.
36. Gunstad J, Suhr JA. Cognitive factors in postconcussion syndrome symptom report. Arch Clin Neuropsychol 2004;19(3):391–405.
37. Hoge CW, McGurk D, Castro CA. Cumulative effects associated with recurrent concussion in collegiate football players: the NCAA concussion study. Mild traumatic brain injury in U.S. soldiers returning from Iraq. N Engl J Med 2008;358(5): 113–6.
38. Lees-haley PR, Brown RS. Neuropsychological complaint base rates of 170 personal injury claimants. Arch Clin Neuropsychol 1993;8:203–9.
39. Lees-Haley PR, Fox DD, Courtney JC. A comparison of complaints by mild brain injury claimants and other claimants describing subjective experiences immediately following their injury. Arch Clin Neuropsychol 2001;16(7):689–95.
40. Schneiderman AI, Braver ER, Kang HK. Understanding sequelae of injury mechanisms and mild traumatic brain injury incurred during the conflicts in Iraq and Afghanistan: persistent postconcussive symptoms and posttraumatic stress disorder. Am J Epidemiol 2008;167(12):1446–52.
41. Wang Y, Chan RCK, Deng Y. Examination of postconcussion-like symptoms in healthy university students: relationships to subjective and objective neuropsychological function performance. Arch Clin Neuropsychol 2006;21(4):339–47.
42. Hylin MJ, Orsi Sa, Rozas NS, et al. Repeated mild closed head injury impairs short-term visuospatial memory and complex learning. J Neurotrauma 2013; 30(9):716–26.

43. Luo J, Nguyen A, Villeda S, et al. Long-term cognitive impairments and pathological alterations in a mouse model of repetitive mild traumatic brain injury. Front
Neurol 2014;5:12.

44. Vagnozzi R, Signoretti S, Tavazzi B, et al. Temporal window of metabolic brain
vulnerability to concussion: a pilot 1H-magnetic resonance spectroscopic study
in concussed athletes–part III. Neurosurgery 2008;62(6):1286.

45. Belanger HG, Spiegel E, Vanderploeg RD. Neuropsychological performance
following a history of multiple self-reported concussions: a meta-analysis. J Int
Neuropsychol Soc 2010;16(2):262–7.

46. Iverson GL, Echemendia RJ, LaMarre AK, et al. Possible lingering effects of
multiple past concussions. Rehabil Res Pract 2012;2012:1–7.

47. Connery AK, Baker DA, Kirk JW, et al. The effects of multiple mild traumatic brain
injuries on acute injury presentation and neuropsychological recovery in children.
Neurosurgery 2014;75(1):31–6.

48. Iverson GL, Brooks BL, Lovell MR, et al. No cumulative effects for one or two
previous concussions. Br J Sports Med 2006;40(1):72–5.

49. Randolph C, Kirkwood MW. What are the real risks of sport-related concussion,
and are they modifiable? J Int Neuropsychol Soc 2009;15(4):512–20.

50. Randolph C. Baseline neuropsychological testing in managing sport-related
concussion: does it modify risk? Curr Sports Med Rep 2011;10(1):21–6.

51. Kutcher JS, Eckner JT. At-risk populations in sports-related concussion.
Curr Sports Med Rep 2010;9(1):16–20.

52. Scopaz KA, Hatzenbuehler JR. Risk modifiers for concussion and prolonged
recovery. Sports Health 2013;5(6):537–41.

53. Makdissi M, Davis G, Jordan B, et al. Revisiting the modifiers: how should the
evaluation and management of acute concussions differ in specific groups?
Br J Sports Med 2013;47(5):314–20.

54. Meehan WP, Taylor AM, Proctor M. The pediatric athlete: younger athletes with
sport-related concussion. Clin Sports Med 2011;30(1):133–44, x.

55. DiFiori JP, Benjamin HJ, Brenner J, et al. Overuse injuries and burnout in
youth sports: a position statement from the American Medical Society for Sports
Medicine. Clin J Sport Med 2014;24(1):3–20.

56. Halstead ME, Walter KD, Council on Sports Medicine and Fitness. American
Academy of Pediatrics. Clinical report–sport-related concussion in children and
adolescents. Pediatrics 2010;126(3):597–615.

57. Eisenberg MA, Andrea J, Meehan W, et al. Time interval between concussions
and symptom duration. Pediatrics 2013;132(1):8–17.

58. Ellis MJ, Leiter J, Hall T, et al. Neuroimaging findings in pediatric sports-related
concussion. J Neurosurg Pediatr 2015;16(3):241–7.

59. Vassilyadi M, Macartney G, Barrowman N, et al. Symptom experience and quality
of life in children after sport-related head injuries: a cross-sectional study. Pediatr
Neurosurg 2015;50(4):196–203.

60. Yeates KO, Kaizar E, Rusin J, et al. Reliable change in postconcussive symptoms
and its functional consequences among children with mild traumatic brain injury.
Arch Pediatr Adolesc Med 2012;166(7):615–22.

61. DiFazio M, Silverberg ND, Kirkwood MW, et al. Prolonged activity restriction after
concussion: are we worsening outcomes? Clin Pediatr (Phila) 2015. [Epub ahead
of print].

62. Laker SR. Sports-related concussion. Curr Pain Headache Rep 2015;19(8):41.

Potential Long-Term Consequences of Concussive and Subconcussive Injury

Bertrand R. Huber, MD, PhD[a,b], Michael L. Alosco, PhD[c],
Thor D. Stein, MD, PhD[a,c,d,e], Ann C. McKee, MD[a,b,c,d,*]

KEYWORDS

- Neuropathology • Trauma • Traumatic brain injury
- Chronic traumatic encephalopathy • Tau • Concussion • Subconcussion

KEY POINTS

- Individuals with a history of repetitive head impacts are at risk for developing chronic traumatic encephalopathy (CTE).
- CTE is a unique neurodegenerative disorder characterized by perivascular deposits of hyperphosphorylated tau at the depths of the cerebral sulci.
- The number of years of exposure to contact sports, not the number of concussions, is significantly associated with more severe tau abnormality in CTE, suggesting that repetitive head trauma, including subconcussive injury, is the primary driver of disease.
- Recent studies in neurodegenerative disease brain bank cohorts suggest that changes of CTE are relatively common.

Over the last decade, there has been considerable interest in the potential long-term effects of concussive and subconcussive injury that occur in association with the play of contact sports. Case reports and case series have described athletes who developed explosivity, loss of control, aggressive and violent behaviors, impaired attention,

Disclosures: None.
[a] VA Boston HealthCare System, 150 South Huntington Avenue, Boston, MA 02130, USA;
[b] Department of Neurology, Boston University School of Medicine, 72 East Concord Street, B-7800, Boston, MA 02118, USA; [c] Chronic Traumatic Encephalopathy Program, Boston University School of Medicine, 72 East Concord Street, B-7800, Boston, MA 02118, USA; [d] Department of Pathology, Boston University School of Medicine, 72 East Concord Street, B-7800, Boston, MA 02118, USA; [e] Bedford Veterans Affairs Medical Center, 200 Springs Road, Building 18, Room 118, Bedford, MA 01730, USA
* Corresponding author. Department of Neurology, Boston University School of Medicine, 72 East Concord Street, B-7800, Boston, MA 02118.
E-mail address: amckee@bu.edu

Phys Med Rehabil Clin N Am 27 (2016) 503–511
http://dx.doi.org/10.1016/j.pmr.2015.12.007
1047-9651/16/$ – see front matter Published by Elsevier Inc.
pmr.theclinics.com

depression, executive dysfunction, and memory disturbances associated with chronic traumatic encephalopathy (CTE). There have been debates about how commonly CTE occurs, whether CTE is a distinct neurodegeneration, and if the repetitive head impacts that occur during the play of sports are causal to CTE development. The disease symptoms lack specificity, and the absence of longitudinal, prospective clinical studies with neuropathologic analysis limits understanding of the full clinical spectrum. However, current data indicate that the neuropathology of CTE is unique and can be readily distinguished from other neurodegenerative diseases; that exposure to repetitive head impacts, not the number of concussions, is the primary driver of CTE abnormality; and that CTE is more common than currently recognized.

The variety of clinical symptoms associated with boxing was first described by Harrison Martland[1] in 1928, who found abnormalities in "nearly one half of the fighters who stayed in the game long enough."[1] The general public referred to the condition as "punch drunk," "goofy," and "slug-nutty,"[2,3] and later the terms "dementia pugilistica"[4] and "chronic traumatic encephalopathy" or "CTE" were introduced.[5] Over the intervening decades since the recognition of CTE, clinical and neuropathologic evidence has emerged indicating that CTE occurs in association with American football, boxing, wrestling, ice hockey, baseball, and soccer. CTE has also been associated with other forms of mild repetitive head injury, such as physical abuse, epileptic seizures, head banging, and activities related to military service.[6–12]

CLINICAL SIGNS AND SYMPTOMS OF CHRONIC TRAUMATIC ENCEPHALOPATHY

The clinical symptoms of CTE typically develop insidiously, years to decades after exposure to repetitive brain trauma, and progress slowly over years to decades.[13–15] Occasionally, persistent symptoms develop while an individual is still active in a sport that may be difficult to distinguish from prolonged post-concussive syndrome.[16] In the authors' series of 119 neuropathologically confirmed CTE cases, the mean age at symptom onset was 44.3 years (standard error of the mean [SEM] = 1.5, range 16–83 years), 14.5 years after retirement from the sport (SEM = 1.6, n = 104). However, 22% of individuals later diagnosed with CTE were symptomatic at the time of retirement. The clinical course is often protracted (mean duration = 15.0 years, SEM = 1.2, n = 125).[14,17,18] It is unclear what factors mitigate the wide age range of clinical onset, and many are the focus of current research investigation. Genetics may play a role in an individual's relative susceptibility or resistance to the adverse effects of repetitive neurotrauma and factors such as cognitive reserve, including educational attainment and environmental enrichment, and age at first exposure may influence the clinical expression of the disease.

The clinical presentation of CTE characteristically begins in one or more of 4 distinct domains: mood, behavior, cognitive, and motor. Early behavioral symptoms include explosivity, verbal and physical violence, loss of control, impulsivity, paranoia, and rage behaviors.[15,19] Cognitively, the most prominent deficits are memory, executive functioning, and impaired attention. Approximately 45% of subjects with CTE develop dementia; of subjects older than the age of 60 years, 66% develop dementia. Complaints of chronic headaches occur in 30%[15]; motor symptoms, including dysarthria, dysphagia, coordination problems, and parkinsonism (tremor, decreased facial expression, rigidity, and gait instability), may also develop.[20]

Stern and colleagues[15] distinguished 2 courses of clinical presentation. The first type presents with mood and behavioral symptoms early in life (mean age = 35 years) and progresses in severity to include cognitive symptoms later in the disease course. The second course presents with cognitive symptoms later in life (mean age = 60 years) and often progresses to also include mood and behavioral symptoms.

CLINICAL DIAGNOSIS OF CHRONIC TRAUMATIC ENCEPHALOPATHY

Like many neurodegenerative diseases, the current lack of available biomarkers for CTE precludes a definitive diagnosis during life, and the disease can only be diagnosed definitively at postmortem examination. Three groups have proposed preliminary diagnostic criteria for the clinical diagnosis of CTE.[19,21,22]

The proposed criteria differentiate between possible and probable CTE based on various clinical symptoms and follow a structure similar to the National Institute on Aging-Alzheimer's Association clinical diagnostic criteria for other neurodegenerative diseases.[23] The criteria of Montenigro and colleagues[19] distinguish between the clinical syndrome of CTE, referred to as Traumatic Encephalopathy Syndrome (TES), and the pathologic diagnosis of CTE, which is reserved for postmortem diagnosis. The TES syndrome is dichotomized into subtypes based on the presence or absence of various groups of symptoms, including Behavioral/Mood Variant, Cognitive Variant, Mixed Variant, and TES Dementia (for a full review, see Montenigro and colleagues[19]).

Whether the proposed clinical criteria are able to differentiate CTE from other abnormalities with a high degree of sensitivity and specificity in both research and clinical settings has not been determined.

Ongoing large-scale retrospective studies, such as the recently funded Understanding Neurologic Injury and Traumatic Encephalopathy (UNITE) UO1 project from the National Institute of Neurological Disease and Stroke (NINDS) and the National Institute of Biomedical Imaging and Bioengineering (NIBIB), examines the clinical presentation of brain donors designated as "at risk" for the development of CTE, develops a blinded consensus clinical diagnosis, and compares the clinical consensus diagnosis to equally blinded postmortem neuropathologic assessment.[24] Preliminary indications are that the clinical criteria for CTE are highly sensitive but lack specificity.[25] Additional analyses using data from the UNITE study will provide detailed information on the specificity of item-level symptoms to allow further refinements in the clinical criteria. To date, nearly all information collected regarding the clinical presentation of CTE has come from retrospective analysis of subjects analyzed after death.[14,15] Recent funding of large-scale longitudinal prospective studies will also help clarify the precise clinical distinctions between CTE and other neurodegenerative and neuropsychiatric disorders.

BIOMARKERS

The use of in vivo biomarkers could greatly improve the accurate clinical diagnosis of CTE as well as facilitate the monitoring of disease progression and the efficacy of disease-modifying therapies. Although no diagnostic biomarkers are currently available, several promising techniques are being developed. Tau-specific PET ligands have demonstrated encouraging results in Alzheimer disease (AD)[26,27] and detect the progression of AD tauopathy among individuals along the cognitive spectrum.[28] Studies using diffusion tensor imaging have also showed promise in their ability to detect changes to white matter integrity following head trauma.[29] In addition, functional connectivity (functional MRI [fMRI]) and other advanced imaging measures of axonal integrity, such as magnetic resonance spectroscopy, to detect biochemical metabolites as well as cerebrospinal fluid and plasma protein markers (including p-tau and total tau) are all under investigation.[23,30,31]

NEUROPATHOLOGY OF CHRONIC TRAUMATIC ENCEPHALOPATHY
Gross Abnormality

Grossly identifiable changes are usually minimal in the early stages of CTE; in advanced disease, there is often reduced brain weight, cerebral atrophy that is typically most severe in the frontal and anterior temporal lobes, enlargement of the lateral and third ventricles, cavum septum pellucidum with fenestrations, thinning of the corpus callosum, atrophy of the diencephalon and mammillary bodies, and depigmentation of the locus coeruleus and substantia nigra. Cerebellar scarring was commonly reported in the early reports of CTE in boxers; however, grossly identifiable cerebellar abnormalities are rarely present in CTE associated with football or other sports.[14]

Microscopic Abnormality

CTE is a tauopathy and is characterized by the deposition of hyperphosphorylated tau (p-tau) protein as neurofibrillary tangles NFTs, thorned astrocytes (TA), and neurites in a unique pattern in the brain. The tau pathology is characteristically perivascular in distribution and shows a predilection for the depths of the cerebral sulci. In 2013, McKee and colleagues[14] described a spectrum of p-tau abnormality in 68 male subjects with a history of exposure to repetitive brain trauma with neuropathologic evidence of CTE, ranging in age from 17 to 98 years (mean 59.5 years) and proposed provisional criteria for neuropathologic diagnosis. In young subjects with the mildest forms of CTE, focal perivascular epicenters of NFTs and TA were found clustered at the depths of the neocortical sulci; in subjects with severe disease, there was evidence of a widespread tauopathy with focal concentration of pathology perivascularly at the sulcal depths and in the superficial cortical layers. Other abnormalities encountered in advanced CTE include abnormal deposits of phosphorylated TAR DNA-binding protein of 43-kDa (TDP-43) protein that occasionally colocalizes with p-tau, and varying degrees of Aβ abnormality, axonal dystrophy, and neuroinflammation.[14,32]

Recently, as the first part of a series of consensus panels funded by the NINDS/NIBIB to define the neuropathologic criteria for CTE, the McKee neuropathologic criteria were used by 7 neuropathologists to evaluate 25 cases of various tauopathies, including CTE, AD, progressive supranuclear palsy, argyrophilic grain disease, corticobasal degeneration, primary age-related tauopathy, and parkinsonism dementia complex of Guam. The neuropathologists evaluated the cases blinded to all information on age, gender, clinical symptoms, diagnosis, athletic exposure, and gross neuropathologic findings and determined that there was good agreement between reviewers and the diagnosis of CTE (Cohen's kappa: 0.78) and excellent identification of the cases of CTE. Based on these results, the panel refined the diagnostic pathologic criteria for CTE and defined a pathognomonic lesion. The lesion considered pathognomonic for CTE is an accumulation of abnormal tau in neurons and astroglia distributed around small blood vessels at the depths of cortical sulci and in an irregular pattern. The panel also defined supportive but nonspecific features of CTE.[33]

Staging of Chronic Traumatic Encephalopathy

McKee and colleagues[14] also described 4 distinct stages of CTE, defined by the extent of the tau abnormalities. Stage I CTE is characterized by isolated perivascular foci of p-tau as NFTs and TA at the sulcal depths of the cerebral cortex. In stage II CTE, multiple foci of p-tau are found in the cerebral cortices. In stage III CTE, NFT are found in the superficial cortices adjacent to the focal epicenters, and there is involvement of the medial temporal lobe structures (hippocampus, amygdala, entorhinal cortex). In stage IV CTE, there is severe widespread p-tau pathology in the cortices, diencephalon, brainstem, and cerebellum (reviewed in McKee and colleagues[14]). Furthermore, among former American football players, the stage of CTE severity correlates significantly with the duration of exposure to football, age at death, and years since retirement from football.[14]

Recently, 2 large academic centers have reported comorbid CTE changes in their neurodegenerative disease brain banks.[34,35] In the brain bank series reported by Bieniek and colleagues,[34] 21 of 66 (31.8%) former athletes had cortical tau abnormalities consistent with CTE on postmortem neuropathologic examination. Moreover, CTE pathology was not detected in 198 individuals who had no exposure to contact sports, including 33 individuals with documented single-incident traumatic brain injury sustained from falls, motor vehicle accidents, domestic violence, or assaults. Ling and colleagues[35] found the occurrence of CTE in 11.9% of 268 screened cases of neurodegenerative diseases and controls.

Relationship of Tau Abnormality to Trauma

Although CTE is associated with repetitive head impacts, the pathophysiological mechanisms critical to developing a progressive tauopathy after repetitive trauma are only beginning to be identified. Traumatic axonal injury results in alterations in axonal membrane permeability, ionic shifts including massive influx of calcium, and release of caspases and calpains that trigger tau phosphorylation, misfolding, truncation, and aggregation, as well as breakdown of the cytoskeleton with dissolution of microtubules and neurofilaments.[36–38] Acceleration and deceleration forces on the brain, rotational as well as linear, cause the brain to elongate and deform. These shearing forces predominantly affect long fibers, specifically axons and blood vessels,[39,40] and are typically most severe at the depths of the cerebral sulci and at the interface between brain parenchyma and cerebral vasculature.[41] The irregular distribution of the p-tau abnormality in the perivascular region and sulcal depths of the neocortex corresponds to these areas of greatest tissue displacement. In addition, the early and predominant involvement of the superior and dorsolateral frontal lobes in former football players parallels the high frequency of impacts to the top of the head compared with those to the front, back, and side of the head in football players,[42,43] as well as fMRI data showing activation impairments in dorsolateral prefrontal cortex that is associated with significantly higher numbers of head collisions to the top-front of the head.[44]

Increasing evidence indicates that tau phosphorylation, truncation, aggregation, and polymerization into filaments represent a toxic gain of function, and continued accumulation of p-tau leads to neurodegeneration. This finding is supported by tau's involvement in some genetic forms of frontotemporal degeneration[45] and by work that shows that plasmids containing human tau complementary DNA constructs microinjected into lamprey neurons in situ produce tau filaments that accumulate and lead to neuronal degeneration.[46,47] However, it is also possible that the intracellular NFTs are the byproducts rather than the cause of cellular injury and that NFT formation indicates neurons that survived the initial injury and sequestered the abnormally phosphorylated, truncated, and folded tau.[48]

β-Amyloid

β-Amyloid (Aβ) plaques are found in 52% of individuals with CTE,[18] in contrast to the extensive Aβ plaques that characterize nearly all cases of AD. Although Aβ plaques are typically abundant in AD and are essential to the diagnosis, Aβ plaques in CTE, when they occur, are less dense and predominantly diffuse.[7] In CTE, Aβ plaques are significantly associated with accelerated tauopathy, Lewy body formation, dementia, parkinsonism, and inheritance of the ApoE4 allele.[18]

TDP-43

TDP-43 proteinopathy is also found in approximately 80% of subjects with CTE.[8] Moreover, some athletes with CTE also develop a motor neuron disease that is clinically indistinguishable from amyotrophic lateral sclerosis.[8] The presence of multiple abnormally aggregated phosphorylated proteins in CTE suggests that a common stimulus, such as repetitive trauma, provokes the accumulation of neurodegenerative proteins or that the presence of p-tau aggregates provokes the accumulation of other pathologic proteins such as Aß and TDP-43.[49] TDP-43 plays a critical role in mediating the response of the neuronal cytoskeleton to axonal injury by virtue of its capacity to bind to neurofilament messenger RNA (mRNA) and stabilize the mRNA transcript. TDP-43 is also intrinsically prone to aggregation and its expression is upregulated after experimental axotomy.[50] Traumatic axotomy may accelerate TDP-43 accumulation, aggregation, and dislocation to the cytoplasm, and enhance its neurotoxicity.

RISK AND PROTECTIVE FACTORS

There are many potential variables surrounding exposure to repetitive head impacts that might influence the risk for CTE later in life. The age at which athletes experience head impacts may influence CTE risk. Recent studies in retired National Football League athletes indicate that exposure to football before the age of 12 is associated with greater cognitive impairment and more white matter abnormalities on MRI.[51,52] It remains to be determined what other lifestyle factors might mitigate the risk for CTE. Chronic inflammation, such as accompanies obesity, hypertension, diabetes mellitus, atherosclerosis, and heart disease, may facilitate neurodegeneration and NFT formation.[53–56] In contrast, greater cognitive reserve might lessen or delay the development of clinical symptoms in CTE. Genetic variations are also likely to play an important role in moderating the relationships between exposure to head trauma, neuropathologic changes, and disordered cognition and behavior. A recent study indicated a slight increase in *MAPT* H1 haplotype in subjects with sports exposure and CTE abnormality compared with those without CTE abnormality.[34]

SUMMARY

CTE is a neurodegenerative disease that occurs after exposure to repetitive head trauma. CTE has been reported in association with American football, wrestling, soccer, ice hockey, rugby, physical abuse, poorly controlled epilepsy, head banging behaviors, and military service, suggesting that trauma of diverse origin is capable of instigating CTE. Cumulative exposure to trauma, not the number of concussions, is associated with the severity of p-tau abnormality, suggesting that subconcussive impacts are an important driver of disease. CTE most commonly manifests in midlife and produces clinical symptoms of disordered cognition, memory loss and executive dysfunction, depression, apathy, disinhibition, and irritability, as well as parkinsonism. The neuropathology of CTE is increasingly well defined; a NINDs/NIBIB panel of expert neuropathologists has defined preliminary criteria and a pathognomonic lesion for the neuropathologic diagnosis of CTE. Currently, neuropathologic examination of brain tissue is the only way to diagnose CTE, although intense research efforts are underway to identify biomarkers to detect and monitor the disease during life and to develop therapies to slow or reverse its course. Newly funded longitudinal, prospective research efforts will shed additional light on critical variables related to head trauma exposure, genetics, and lifestyle factors that influence the development of CTE.

REFERENCES

1. Martland HS. Punch drunk. J Am Med Assoc 1928;91:1103–7.
2. Critchley M. Medical aspects of boxing, particularly from a neurological standpoint. Br Med J 1957;1(5015):357.
3. Parker HL. Traumatic encephalopathy ('punch drunk') of professional pugilists. J Neurol Psychopathol 1934;15(57):20.
4. Millspaugh JA. Dementia pugilistica. U S Nav Med Bull 1937;35:7.
5. Critchley M. Punch drunk syndromes: the chronic traumatic encephalopathy of boxers. In: Hommage à Clovis Vincent. Maloine (Paris): 1949.
6. Geddes JF, Vowles GH, Nicoll JAR, et al. Neuronal cytoskeletal changes are an early consequence of repetitive head injury. Acta Neuropathol 1999;98(2):171–8.
7. McKee AC, Cantu RC, Nowinski CJ, et al. Chronic traumatic encephalopathy in athletes: progressive tauopathy after repetitive head injury. J Neuropathol Exp Neurol 2009;68(7):709–35.
8. McKee AC, Gavett BE, Stern RA, et al. TDPE43 proteinopathy and motor neuron disease in chronic traumatic encephalopathy. J Neuropathol Exp Neurol 2010; 69(9):918–29.
9. Omalu BI, Bailes J, Hammers JL, et al. Chronic traumatic encephalopathy, suicides and parasuicides in professional American athletes the role of the forensic pathologist. Am J Forensic Med Pathol 2010;31(2):130–2.
10. Omalu BI, DeKosky ST, Hamilton RL, et al. Chronic traumatic encephalopathy in a national football league player: part II. Neurosurgery 2006;59(5):1086–92.
11. Omalu BI, DeKosky ST, Minster RL, et al. Chronic traumatic encephalopathy in a National Football League player. Neurosurgery 2005;57(1):128–33.
12. Cajigal S. Brain damage may have contributed to former wrestler's violent demise. Neurol Today 2007;7:16.
13. Corsellis J, Bruton C, Freeman EB, et al. The aftermath of boxing. Psychol Med 1973;3(03):270–303.
14. McKee AC, Stern RA, Nowinski CJ, et al. The spectrum of disease in chronic traumatic encephalopathy. Brain 2013;136(Pt 1):43–64.
15. Stern RA, Daneshvar DH, Baugh CM, et al. Clinical presentation of chronic traumatic encephalopathy. Neurology 2013;81(13):1122–9.
16. Mez J, Solomon T, Daneshvar D, et al. Pathologically confirmed chronic traumatic encephalopathy in a 25 year old former college football player. JAMA Neurology, in press.
17. Stein TD, Alvarez VE, McKee AC. Chronic traumatic encephalopathy: a spectrum of neuropathological changes following repetitive brain trauma in athletes and military personnel. Alzheimers Res Ther 2014;6(1):4.
18. Stein TD, Montenigro PH, Alvarez VE, et al. Beta-amyloid deposition in chronic traumatic encephalopathy. Acta Neuropathol 2015;130(1):21–34.
19. Montenigro PH, Baugh CM, Daneshvar DH, et al. Clinical subtypes of chronic traumatic encephalopathy: literature review and proposed research diagnostic criteria for traumatic encephalopathy syndrome. Alzheimers Res Ther 2014; 6(5–8):1–17.
20. Mez J, Stern RA, McKee AC. Chronic traumatic encephalopathy: where are we and where are we going? Curr Neurol Neurosci Rep 2013;13(12):1–12.

21. Victoroff J. Traumatic encephalopathy: review and provisional research diagnostic criteria. NeuroRehabilitation 2013;32(2):211–24.
22. Jordan BD. The clinical spectrum of sport-related traumatic brain injury. Nature reviews. Neurology 2013;9(4):222–30.
23. McKhann GM, Knopman DS, Chertkow H, et al. The diagnosis of dementia due to Alzheimer's disease: recommendations from the National Institute on Aging-Alzheimer's Association workgroups on diagnostic guidelines for Alzheimer's disease. Alzheimers Demen 2011;7(3):263–9.
24. Mez J, Solomon TM, Daneshvar DH, et al. Assessing clinicopathological correlation in chronic traumatic encephalopathy: rationale and methods for the UNITE study. Alzheimers Res Ther 2015;7(1):1–14.
25. Mez J, Solomon TM, Daneshvar DH, et al. Validity of clinical research criteria for chronic traumatic encephalopathy. Presented at Traumatic Brain Injury: Clinical, Pathological and Translational Mechanisms. Santa Fe (NM), January 24–27, 2016.
26. Xia CEF, Arteaga J, Chen G, et al. [18 F] T807, a novel tau positron emission tomography imaging agent for Alzheimer's disease. Alzheimers Demen 2013;9(6): 666–76.
27. Chien DT, Bahri S, Szardenings AK, et al. Early clinical PET imaging results with the novel PHF-tau radioligand [F-18]-T807. J Alzheimers Dis 2013;34(2):457–68.
28. Johnson KA, Schultz A, Betensky RA, et al. Tau PET imaging in aging and early Alzheimer's disease. Ann Neurol 2015. [Epub ahead of print].
29. Koerte IK, Ertl-Wagner B, Reiser M, et al. White matter integrity in the brains of professional soccer players without a symptomatic concussion. JAMA 2012; 308(18):1859–61.
30. Buerger K, Ewers M, Pirttilä T, et al. CSF phosphorylated tau protein correlates with neocortical neurofibrillary pathology in Alzheimer's disease. Brain 2006; 129(11):3035–41.
31. Lin A, Liao H, Merugumala S, et al. Metabolic imaging of mild traumatic brain injury. Brain Imaging Behav 2012;6(2):208–23.
32. McKee AC, Gavett BE, Stern RA, et al. TDP-43 proteinopathy and motor neuron disease in chronic traumatic encephalopathy. J Neuropathol Exp Neurol 2010; 69(9):918–29.
33. McKee AC, Cairns NJ, Dickson DW, et al. The first NINDS consensus meeting to define neuropathological criteria for the diagnosis of chronic traumatic encephalopathy. Acta Neuropathol 2015. [Epub ahead of print].
34. Bieniek KF, Ross OA, Cormier KA, et al. Chronic traumatic encephalopathy pathology in a neurodegenerative disorders brain bank. Acta Neuropathol 2015; 130(6):877–89.
35. Ling H, Holton JL, Shaw K, et al. Histological evidence of chronic traumatic encephalopathy in a large series of neurodegenerative diseases. Acta Neuropathol 2015. [Epub ahead of print].
36. Binder LI, Guillozet-Bongaarts AL, Garcia-Sierra F, et al. Tau, tangles, and Alzheimer's disease. Biochim Biophys Acta 2005;1739(2–3):216–23.
37. Giza CC, Hovda DA. The neurometabolic cascade of concussion. J Athl Train 2001;36(3):228–35.
38. Serbest G, Burkhardt MF, Siman R, et al. Temporal profiles of cytoskeletal protein loss following traumatic axonal injury in mice. Neurochem Res 2007;32(12): 2006–14.
39. Maxwell WL, Povlishock JT, Graham DL. A mechanistic analysis of nondisruptive axonal injury: a review. J Neurotrauma 1997;14(7):419–40.

40. Medana I, Esiri M. Axonal damage: a key predictor of outcome in human CNS diseases. Brain 2003;126(3):515–30.
41. Cloots R, Van Dommelen J, Nyberg T, et al. Micromechanics of diffuse axonal injury: influence of axonal orientation and anisotropy. Biomech Model Mechanobiol 2011;10(3):413–22.
42. Guskiewicz KM, Mihalik JP, Shankar V, et al. Measurement of head impacts in collegiate football players: relationship between head impact biomechanics and acute clinical outcome after concussion. Neurosurgery 2007;61(6):1244–53.
43. Mihalik JP, Bell DR, Marshall SW, et al. Measurement of head impacts in collegiate football players: an investigation of positional and event-type differences. Neurosurgery 2007;61(6):1229–35.
44. Talavage TM, Nauman EA, Breedlove EL, et al. Functionally-detected cognitive impairment in high school football players without clinically-diagnosed concussion. J Neurotrauma 2014;31(4):327–38.
45. Spillantini MG, Bird TD, Ghetti B. Frontotemporal dementia and parkinsonism linked to chromosome 17: a new group of tauopathies. Brain Pathol 1998;8(2): 387–402.
46. Hall GF, Chu BY, Lee G, et al. Human tau filaments induce microtubule and synapse loss in an in vivo model of neurofibrillary degenerative disease. J Cell Sci 2000;113(8):1373–87.
47. Hall GF, Yao J, Lee G. Human tau becomes phosphorylated and forms filamentous deposits when overexpressed in lamprey central neurons in situ. Proc Natl Acad Sci U S A 1997;94(9):4733–8.
48. de Calignon A, Fox LM, Pitstick R, et al. Caspase activation precedes and leads to tangles. Nature 2010;464(7292):1201–4.
49. Uryu K, Chen XH, Martinez D, et al. Multiple proteins implicated in neurodegenerative diseases accumulate in axons after brain trauma in humans. Exp Neurol 2007;208(2):185–92.
50. Moisse K, Mepham J, Volkening K, et al. Cytosolic TDP-43 expression following axotomy is associated with caspase 3 activation in NFL-/- mice: support for a role for TDP-43 in the physiological response to neuronal injury. Brain Res 2009;1296:176–86.
51. Stamm JM, Bourlas AP, Baugh CM, et al. Age of first exposure to football and later-life cognitive impairment in former NFL players. Neurology 2015;84(11): 1114–20.
52. Stamm JM, Koerte IK, Muehlmann M, et al. Age at first exposure to football is associated with altered corpus callosum white matter microstructure in former professional football players. J Neurotrauma 2015;32(22):1768–76.
53. Arnaud L, Robakis NK, Figueiredo-Pereira ME. It may take inflammation, phosphorylation and ubiquitination to 'tangle' in Alzheimer's disease. Neurodegener Dis 2006;3(6):313–9.
54. Arnaud LT, Myeku N, Figueiredo-Pereira ME. Proteasome-caspase-cathepsin sequence leading to tau pathology induced by prostaglandin J2 in neuronal cells. J Neurochem 2009;110(1):328–42.
55. Duong TH, Nikolaeva M, Acton PJ. C-reactive protein-like immunoreactivity in the neurofibrillary tangles of Alzheimer's disease. Brain Res 1997;749(1):152–6.
56. Ke YD, Delerue F, Gladbach A, et al. Experimental diabetes mellitus exacerbates tau pathology in a transgenic mouse model of Alzheimer's disease. PLoS One 2009;4(11):e7917.

Effects of Legislation on Sports-Related Concussion

Leah G. Concannon, MD

KEYWORDS

- Concussion • Legislation • Athletics • Sports

KEY POINTS

- Current concussion legislation centers on the following three points: Education of athletes, parents, and coaches; removal from practice or play for suspected concussion; and clearance by a health care provider before medically supervised graded return to play.
- Sports concussion laws are not designed for primary prevention but instead aid in proper diagnosis and management after an injury has occurred, thereby preventing the tragedies that may occur from premature return to play.
- Laws are living documents and can be amended as more research becomes available.

INTRODUCTION

Although public knowledge and awareness of concussions has increased over the years, it is estimated that before 2009, up to 40% of concussed youth athletes were prematurely returned to play after concussions.[1] This premature return to play is widely thought to have led to tragic results, as one study found that 71% of football players that suffered a catastrophic head injury received a previous concussion in the same season, and 39% were playing with residual symptoms from a concussion.[2] Despite multiple published guidelines and educational campaigns, tragedies still occur in youth sports after concussions.

The national push for concussion legislation began with the story of one child. Zackery Lystedt was 13 years old when, in 2006, he suffered a concussion while playing in a middle school football game. When Zack was holding his head and slow to get up after a tackle, an injury timeout was called and he was assessed by his coach. No medical personnel was on the sideline, as is typical in many middle school games. Zack sat out the next 2 plays until halftime and returned to play in the third quarter. He had increasing symptoms but continued to play, only to collapse in his father's arms after the game was over. He was airlifted to a level 1 trauma center, where he received

The author has no conflicts of interest.

Division of Sports and Spine, Department of Rehabilitation Medicine, University of Washington, 325 9th Avenue, Box 359721, Seattle, WA 98104, USA

E-mail address: lgconcan@uw.edu

craniotomies for bilateral subdural hematomas. Zack's road to recovery has been long and incomplete, as he continues to struggle daily with cognitive impairments and spastic hemiplegia.

As the Lystedt family labored to find meaning in this injury, they were assisted by their attorney, Richard Adler, president of the Brain Injury Alliance of Washington at the time. Efforts to initiate change in concussion management began first with a state-wide education program. This program was accomplished with help from the local National Football League team (Seattle Seahawks), one of their physicians (Dr Stanley Herring), and the Centers for Disease Control and Prevention (CDC) Heads Up concussion education and awareness program. However, it became apparent that education alone was not enough. Adler describes an "inconsistency gap" that remains even after education; coaches continued to have different levels of understanding surrounding concussion, and many did not recognize the seriousness of a brain injury.[3]

Another issue is the lack of institutional memory.[4] One coach or one athletic director may be well educated in concussion management, but when that individual leaves a program or a school, strategies and policies fail to remain in place, as they have not become institutionalized into the culture of the school or school district. The result is that different schools or school districts may have different policies regarding concussions. In this respect, some athletes may therefore be safer than other athletes. Additionally, the conclusion was reached that education alone does not change behavior, and only legislation combined with the educational effort would help make concussion awareness and management more uniform.

With help from the Brain Injury Alliance of Washington, The University of Washington, the Washington State Athletic Trainers' Association, the Washington Interscholastic Activities Association, and many others, Washington State's Engrossed House Bill 1824 (Zackery Lystedt Law)[5] was passed unanimously on May 14, 2009. By January 2014, less than 5 years later, all 50 states and the District of Columbia had also adopted youth sports concussion laws.[6] To put this in perspective, only 21 states require bicycle helmets for all children, and only 34 have a primary seat belt law.[7]

Sports concussion laws are not designed for primary prevention but instead aid in proper diagnosis and management after an injury has occurred, thereby preventing the tragedies that may occur from premature return to play. To effect this, the Lystedt Law has 3 basic tenets[5]:

1. Education of athletes, parents, and coaches
2. Removal from practice or play for a suspected concussion at the time of the suspected injury
3. Medically supervised return to play

With the exception of Wyoming, the laws in all other states and the District of Columbia also stipulate these 3 tenets.[8] Wyoming only requires establishing protocols for education of coaches and athletic trainers (without specifying requirements) and to address restrictions from school events after suffering a concussion.[9] It does not require removal of athletes from games or practices if they are suspected to have suffered a concussion, nor does it require medical clearance before return to play. For the purposes of this article, the term *sports concussion law* will be used to indicate adherence to these 3 tenets.

EDUCATION

The first tenet of sports concussion laws is education of athletes, parents, and coaches. However, it is generally not specified how this education should occur.

Implementation of educational programs for families and coaches is, therefore, somewhat variable. The Lystedt Law requires that, at a minimum, "on a yearly basis, a concussion and head injury information sheet shall be signed and returned by the youth athlete and the athlete's parent and/or guardian prior to the youth athlete's initiating practice or competition."[5]

Additionally, "each school district's board of directors shall work in concert with the Washington interscholastic activities association (WIAA) to develop the guidelines and other pertinent information and forms to inform and educate coaches, youth athletes, and their parents and/or guardians of the nature and risk of concussion and head injury including continuing to play after concussion or head injury."[5] Many other states have taken a similar route by requiring education of coaches but without stipulating the specifics of how it should occur. This task is often given over to a statewide sports governing body. As will be discussed later, the Lystedt Law, as written, does not directly mandate education of coaches. This is true in many other states as well, whereas some have explicitly mandated annual education of coaches.

REMOVAL FROM PLAY

In keeping with the provisions of the Lystedt Law, "a youth athlete who is suspected of sustaining a concussion or head injury in a practice or game shall be removed from competition at that time."[5] Diagnosis and management of concussions is a medical issue, and only a health care provider is expected to evaluate an athlete to determine if a concussion has occurred. Coaches do not have the medical training to diagnose concussions and are not expected to do so. By stipulating that any athlete *suspected* of a concussion is removed from play, coaches need only to recognize when a concussion may have occurred and are not expected to rule in or rule out a concussion. Education of coaches often directly highlights the signs and symptoms that indicate a possible concussion and that require removal from play. Immediate removal of an athlete from play helps avoid devastating injuries such as second impact syndrome and subdural hematomas.

RETURN TO PLAY

In Washington, "a youth athlete who has been removed from play may not return to play until the athlete is evaluated by a licensed health care provider trained in the evaluation and management of concussion and receives written clearance to return to play from that health care provider."[5] In Washington, the WIAA, as the governing body for most interscholastic activities, determined which medical providers it would accept as qualified to make return-to-play decisions. This action helped avoid debates about scope of practice during the legislative process, which may have slowed down passage of the law. In states that have specified which providers may provide clearance, contentious battles among provider types have been encountered during the legislative process.[10] In rural areas, access to physicians may be limited. Therefore, it is important to identify other providers that can appropriately manage athletes in a timely fashion, allowing greater access to care and limiting potentially unnecessary restrictions to athletes. Although specific return-to-play guidelines are not specified in the law, the standard of care is a stepwise process that has been thoroughly discussed elsewhere, with at least 24 hours between each step.[11]

CHALLENGES IN EDUCATION

Educational initiatives do work to increase concussion knowledge and awareness, but the optimal method of delivery has not yet been elucidated. The CDC launched the Heads Up: Concussion in Youth Sports initiative in 2007. This program is an online toolkit with information for athletes, parents, coaches, and school administrators. There is also a section designed for physicians. This content is freely available on the CDC web site.[12]

After reviewing the CDC Heads Up materials, 82% of high school coaches found the material helpful, and 50% said it changed their views on concussions.[13] A similar study of coaches of youth sports showed that 77% of coaches reported that they were better able to identify athletes that may have suffered a concussion, and 63% reported increased recognition of the seriousness of concussions.[14] However, these findings indicate that 23% of coaches still did not perceive youth concussions as serious, even after reviewing the material.

To be truly effective, any educational initiative must also change athlete and coach behavior. A study in Washington found that for 58% of parents and 30% of athletes, their only concussion education is signing the required information form before the start of the season.[15] It is not yet clear how well this passive form of education assists in transfer of knowledge and, perhaps more importantly, how well this leads to actual changes in behavior. In fact, 1 year after the Lystedt Law, a survey of parents and coaches involved with youth soccer found that more than 90% knew that concussions were serious and could identify neurologic symptoms associated with concussions, but only 85% knew of the Lystedt Law and only 73% knew that written medical clearance was required before return to play.[16]

Nearly all coaches receive multimodal information,[15] and it may be that this method is more beneficial for learning information and for helping change behavior. Multiple other educational initiatives exist to help increase knowledge and awareness in student athletes, from web-based initiatives, to community outreach educators, to personal stories.[17] The goal of these initiatives is to change behavior and encourage reporting of symptoms by alerting athletes to the dangers of concussions.

CHALLENGES IN ATHLETE REPORTING

Several studies found that athletes still do not always report concussion symptoms, even after the passage of legislation.[18–20] A concussion that is not reported cannot be treated effectively. In a study done in Washington state 1 year after implementation of the Lystedt Law, many athletes still stated they would not always report symptoms.[18] Even athletes that can recognize the signs and symptoms of a concussion may be reluctant to report these symptoms to coaches for fear of being removed from play.[18] Three years after passage of the Lystedt Law, 69% of athletes reported playing with symptoms (most commonly headache), and 40% of these athletes reported their coaches were not aware of their symptoms.[19] A prospective study of female youth soccer players in Washington state from 2008 to 2012 found that 59% reported playing with symptoms both before and after the law was passed.[20]

Other studies found that the most common reasons athletes do not report symptoms are not thinking it was serious enough, not wanting to be removed from play, and not wanting to let down teammates and coaches.[21] Athletes also report thinking that they are expected to play through injuries and that because symptoms are sometimes nonspecific, they do not always want to report them to coaches.[18] Studies find conflicting evidence about whether greater knowledge of concussions is associated with improved athlete reporting.[18,21,22] One study of athletes ages 13 to 18 showed that younger athletes were actually more likely to report symptoms,[22] raising the question of whether nonreporting is a learned behavior as athletes feel more pressure to perform. Legislation is one piece of the puzzle, but changing the culture of athlete reporting will likely take ongoing work.

CHALLENGES IN IMPLEMENTATION

Schools and school districts that are regulated by interscholastic athletic associations already have procedures in place for policy implementation and education. For community and recreational leagues, however, their decentralized nature may make educational initiatives and compliance monitoring more challenging.[10] Getting the word out to health care providers also takes time and effort. Three months after passage of the law in Illinois, almost one-third of pediatricians did not know the law existed, although 77% did provide written documentation about return to play guidelines as part of their usual concussion management.[23] Presumably, awareness of the law has increased substantially in the intervening years, although this has not been studied.

COSTS OF IMPLEMENTATION

The Lystedt Law was specifically crafted to be revenue neutral, indicating that there should be no extra cost to any state or local agency or to the school districts to implement the law. This was a key phrase to help the legislative process but is also a key concept for ongoing success of the law. Much of the educational component of the law has already been discussed above. Coaches' education in multiple other subject areas was already required by the WIAA, so concussion education was able to be distributed with delivery systems already in place. Additionally, the informational sheet for athletes and parents/guardians and an educational video for coaches were developed by physicians at the University of Washington, with the help of an educational grant, which allowed both of these materials to be available for free on the WIAA web site. Physicians also volunteer to give in-person talks about concussion at least yearly at the WIAA Coaches School, again tapping into an educational program that was already in place.

Additional educational materials are available for free at multiple sites, most commonly through the CDC Heads Up program. This program now has specific educational materials for coaches, parents, athletes, game officials, school officials, and health care providers, with online training courses for high school coaches, youth coaches, and clinicians.[24,25] The National Federation of State High School Associations also has free training for coaches.[26]

One possible indirect cost of concussion legislation is that some schools or school districts may choose to have athletic trainers at practices and games of particularly high-risk sports as a response to legislation, but this is generally not mandated by the law. The presence of an athletic trainer helps ensure the health and safety of the athletes for any medical emergency that may occur, not just concussions, and is therefore a likely worthwhile cost.

HEALTH CARE UTILIZATION

The law stipulates that athletes must receive clearance from a medical provider before return to play. It is presumed that this would lead to increased health care costs as well. With passage of the Lystedt Law in Washington State, a partnership was formed with the children's hospital and the only level 1 trauma center in the state to ensure that even children without health care insurance could be seen and evaluated for concussions. With the interim passage of the Affordable Health Care Act, many more children now have health care insurance, thereby enhancing access to providers.

A study by Gibson and colleagues[27] looked at health care utilization from 2006 to June 2012. Not all states had passed concussion legislation by this point, so comparisons between states could be made. They found that concussion-related health care utilization increased in all states after 2009 and increased by only 10% more in those states with legislation as opposed to those without. Even before institution of the Lystedt Law in Washington State, there was a nationwide upward trend in concussion-related health care utilization, and up to 60% of the increase seen after 2009 in those states without legislation is a continuation of that trend. The remainder is thought to be owing to elevated awareness after passage of the law. Interestingly, the rate of concussions seen in Emergency Departments and use of computed tomography scans did not increase, which would appear to indicate that athletes were seeking care through the appropriate channels in outpatient clinics.

Athletes seen for concussions may also incur increased orders for blood work, brain MRI, physical therapy, referrals to specialists, and neuropsychological testing. All of these lead to increased costs for families and insurers. Although many would argue that the increase in health care utilization is appropriate, as it indicates that athletes are now receiving reasonable and necessary medical care for their brain injuries, the financial effects that occur cannot be denied. Additionally, athletes that were merely suspected of suffering a concussion will also require a visit with a health care provider, and some of these athletes may not even have a concussion diagnosed after evaluation, again adding to the cost to the family.

LEGAL LIABILITY

There was concern that having a law in place would increase liability for those taking care of athletes. Instead, however, it helps decrease liability by clarifying the standard of care. The first Consensus Statement in 2002[28] recommended removal from play after a concussion, no same day return to play, and a medically supervised graded return to play after symptom resolution. The prevailing standard of care had, therefore, already been set long before the Lystedt Law came into being. Before the law, different school districts had variable protocols for managing concussions. By limiting variability, the law decreases risk, provided the law is followed.

Additionally, the Lystedt Law and the laws in several other states have liability limitations written into the law to provide protection for volunteers taking care of athletes. These limitations are in the form of either protection from or immunity to lawsuits in the event of an athlete's death or injury as a result of return to play if the laws were correctly followed.[29] Individuals can still be liable in cases of gross negligence or willful misconduct.[5] Good Samaritan laws vary from state to state and may not apply to volunteer physicians, particular if any type of compensation, even nonmonetary, has been received for services. Physicians providing volunteer services are advised to be aware of the specifics of their state's laws.

No penalties are written into the Lystedt Law for organizations or individuals that fail to comply with the components of the law. In Washington, the WIAA, as the governing agency involved in making rules for school sports, can determine what, if any, penalties should be enforced.[3] Connecticut and Pennsylvania have written penalties into their laws for coaches or schools that fail to abide by the components of the law.[30,31]

VARIATIONS ACROSS STATES

Although every state except Wyoming, as described above, adheres to the 3 basic tenets of the Lystedt Law, there is variability from state to state. As has already been stated, the content of the education required is not stipulated in the laws and is, therefore, variable in its implementation. Additionally, not all states require athlete, parent, and coach education.[32] Even in the Lystedt Law, the wording requires a yearly informational sheet for athletes and parents/guardians but only requires that the WIAA develop guidelines and information for coaches' education, without mandating annual education as other states have done.[5] Some states outline specifically those categories of health care providers that can provide clearance for return to play,[29] and in some of these states only physicians can provide clearance.[33] In other states, as in Washington, a specific organization is given the task of determining which providers can provide clearance. Not every state requires that those health care providers that can clear an athlete for return to play must be trained in evaluation and management of concussion,[33] and there is generally no clarification of what training is required. Some states, like Washington, require written clearance before return to play, whereas others only require verbal clearance.[8,33] **Table 1** highlights some of these variabilities. States that are not included in **Table 1** explicitly require athlete, parent, and coach education; removal from play for suspected concussion; and return to play only with written clearance from a medical provider trained in the evaluation and management of concussions. Many states, such as Idaho, Illinois, and Vermont, have amended their initial laws to be more robust and now include the 3 categories discussed above.

Many states have gone above and beyond the 3 tenets of sports concussion laws with interesting additions. Six states (Colorado, Connecticut, Louisiana, Nebraska, New York, Vermont) require that the parent/guardian of the athlete be notified of a suspected concussion.[30,37,47,52,63,64] Four states (Illinois, Nebraska, New Hampshire, Texas) require the parent/guardian to sign a consent form before return to play (this is separate from the informational sheet required before participation).[47,48,59,65] In Utah, the health care provider has to provide a written statement that he/she has completed continuing education on concussion in the last 3 years when they provide the written return to play.[60] New York requires at least 24 hours symptom free before return to play, whereas California and New Mexico require 7 days.[50,52,66] Mississippi outlines in the law that athletes cannot participate in a game until they have done a full practice without return of symptoms.[46] Rhode Island encourages, but does not require, baseline neuropsychological testing and encourages the presence of an athletic trainer at all athletic events.[56] West Virginia requires reporting any suspected concussions to the West Virginia Secondary School Activities Commission, including information on how long it took for return to play.[67] Vermont has many interesting additions including that officials must receive training, coaches must receive training on concussions but also how to teach proper technique to help prevent concussions, the home team must ensure a health care provider is present for all collision sports (football, hockey, lacrosse, wrestling) and are strongly encouraged to do so for all contact sports, and information on all concussions that are sustained must be collected.[64]

Table 1
Key features of sports concussion laws through November 2015

State	Athlete/Parent Education	Coach Education	Removal from Play for Suspected Concussion	Written Clearance for Return to Play	HCP Trained in Concussion Management	Restrictions on HCP That Can Clear an Athlete for Return to Play
AK	X	—	X	X	X	—
AL	X	X	X	X	—	Physician
AZ	X	—	X	X	X	—
CO[a]	X	X	X	X	—	—
DE	X	X	X	X	—	Physician
FL	X	—	X	X	X	—
GA	X	—	X	X	X	—
IA	X	—	X	X	X	—
KS	X	—	X	X	—	—
MA	X	X	X	X	—	—
MO	X	—	X	X	X	—
MS	X	—	X	—	X	—
NE	X	—	X	X	X	—
NH	—	—	X	X	X	—
NM	X	X	X	—	—	—
NV	X	—	X	X	—	—

NY	X	X	X	X	Physician
OH	X	X	X	—	—
OK	X	—	X	X	—
OR	—	X	X	—	—
PA[b]	X	X	X	X	Physician or neuropsychologist
RI	X	X	X	X	Physician
SC	X	—	X	—	Physician
TN[c]	X	X	X	—	Physician or neuropsychologist
TX	X	X	X	—	—
UT	X	—	X	X	—
VA	X	X	X	—	—
WA	X	—	X	X	—
WI	X	—	X	X	—
WY	—	—	—	—	—

Abbreviation: HCP, Health care provider.

[a] CO: Only the neuropsychologist needs to be trained in concussion evaluation and management, other providers do not need to have training.

[b] PA: An athletic trainer can clear an athlete to play only if working under the direction of a physician.

[c] TN: Only the neuropsychologist needs to be trained in concussion evaluation and management, physicians do not need to have training.

Data from Refs. 5,9,31,34–62

CHANGES TO STATE LAWS

Laws are living documents and subject to change as more knowledge is gained surrounding concussions. More than 20 states have already made use of this and enacted changes to their law.[68] There are 3 main areas of change[68]:

1. Expanding coverage of the law
2. Tightening or clarifying existing requirements
3. Introducing efforts at primary prevention

Sports concussion laws specifically cover all youth sports using public land and, therefore, includes some, but not all, private schools and sports clubs. California expanded coverage to include charter and private schools,[66] and Arkansas expanded to recreational sports.[69] New Jersey's law specifically added cheerleading.[70]

Some states clarified what provider types can make return-to-play decisions. Others amended laws to require collection of concussion data or to strengthen the educational components of the law. Four states (Illinois, Nebraska, Virginia, Vermont) added return-to-learn provisions.[61,64,65,71]

Primary prevention is the area of some controversy. Some states have expanded coaches' education to include efforts at reducing hits in practice and games. California instituted a limitation of the number and time of full-contact practices.[72] Although this may indeed be sound practice, there is not enough evidence to recommend specific thresholds for number of impacts.[73]

SUCCESS OF THE LAW

The impetus behind the Lystedt Law, and the laws that followed, was to prevent preventable tragedies after concussion. In each of the 5 years before the implementation of the Lystedt Law, there was a death or subdural hematoma requiring surgery in Washington state during each football season. From 2010 through 2014, there were no deaths or operable subdural hematomas in Washington state.

There was concern that implementation of the law would encourage more athletes to hide their symptoms so they could continue to play. A study of the Seattle public high schools found instead that although the total number of players and total injuries only slightly increased, the number of concussions documented by athletic trainers more than doubled after institution of the Lystedt Law.[74] This finding likely indicates increased awareness of the signs and symptoms of concussions and the importance of reporting symptoms to others. A study of female youth soccer players in Washington found that the proportion of athletes that saw a health care provider (44%) did not change after the passage of the law, but athletes were 2 times more likely have a concussion diagnosed after the law passed.[20]

The literature is still sparse evaluating the effect of legislation in other states. In Rhode Island, compliance with the law is only mandated for schools in the Rhode Island Interscholastic League (a voluntary organization for public and private schools). Although all nonmember schools comply with removal from play and written clearance from a health care provider before return, compliance is higher for member schools with regard to athlete, parent, and coach education.[75]

FUTURE OPPORTUNITIES

Sports concussion laws are living documents and can be modified as new knowledge becomes available. The best method for education of athletes, parents, coaches, and others is not yet determined, but it will likely involve multimodal learning with less passive knowledge transfer. Better educational methods may help to enact a culture of change within organizations. Existing laws can be expanded to ensure all youth athletes are covered. Some have also advocated routinely adding return-to-learn sections to laws.[32] A federal law would help decrease variation among states.

As a result of legislation and increased awareness, youth athletes are now receiving formal diagnoses of concussions at higher rates than before. It is more common now to see younger athletes with a history of 3, 4, or 5 concussions before they even enter high school. Controversy remains over when retirement should be recommended for athletes that have sustained multiple concussions. It is, therefore, important for providers to take a full history of not just the current concussion but any previous concussions to ensure that the athlete has not been overdiagnosed in the past as a result of coaches removing them from play for suspicion of a concussion.

SUMMARY

The Lystedt Law was groundbreaking in its scope and its vision, and its 3 main components have become cornerstones for statewide legislation across the county. The basic principles of concussion management for health care providers have not changed and continue to consist of removal from play after suspected concussion, no same-day return to play, and medically supervised graded return to activity once symptoms have returned to baseline. What has changed is athlete, parent, and coach awareness of concussions and their potentially serious nature. With ongoing efforts to implement new research into best practices and standard of care, the hope is that future tragedies resulting from concussions can be avoided.

REFERENCES

1. Yard EE, Comstock RD. Compliance with return to play guidelines following concussion in US high school athletes, 2005-2008. Brain Inj 2009;23(11):888–98.
2. Boden BP, Tacchetti RL, Cantu RC, et al. Catastrophic head injuries in high school and college football players. Am J Sports Med 2007;35(7):1075–81.
3. Adler RH. Youth sports and concussions: preventing preventable brain injuries. One client, one cause, and a new law. Phys Med Rehabil Clin N Am 2011; 22(4):721–8, ix.
4. Adler RH, Herring SA. Changing the culture of concussion: education meets legislation. PM R 2011;3(10 Suppl 2):S468–70.
5. Washington Certification of Enrollment, Engrossed House Bill 1824. Available at: http://ssl.csg.org/dockets/2011cycle/31B/31Bbills/0531b01bwayouthsportshead injurypolicies.pdf. Accessed August 9, 2015.
6. National Conference of State Legislatures. Available at: http://www.ncsl.org/ research/health/traumatic-brain-injury-legislation.aspx. Accessed September 12, 2015.
7. The Facts Hurt: A State-By-State Injury Prevention Policy Report. Available at: http:// healthyamericans.org/reports/injuryprevention15/. Accessed August 30, 2015.
8. Sports concussion state laws (June 2014). Available at: www.aan.com/practice/ sports-concussion-toolkit/. Accessed September 6, 2015.
9. Wyoming enrolled act 97. Available at: http://legisweb.state.wy.us/2011/Enroll/ SF0038.pdf. Accessed November 1, 2015.
10. Lowrey KM, Morain SR. State experiences implementing youth sports concussion laws: challenges, successes, and lessons for evaluating impact. J Law Med Ethics 2014;42(3):290–6.

11. McCrory P, Meeuwisse WH, Aubry M, et al. Consensus statement on concussion in sport–the 4th International Conference on Concussion in Sport held in Zurich, November 2012. PM R 2013;5(4):255–79.

12. Centers for disease control and prevention. HEADS UP: concussion in youth sports. Available at: http://www.cdc.gov/headsup/youthsports/index.html. Accessed August 16, 2015.

13. Sarmiento K, Mitchko J, Klein C, et al. Evaluation of the Centers for Disease Control and Prevention's concussion initiative for high school coaches: "Heads up: concussion in high school sports. J Sch Health 2010;80(3):112–8.

14. Covassin T, Elbin RJ, Sarmiento K. Educating coaches about concussion in sports: evaluation of the CDC's "heads up: concussion in youth sports" initiative. J Sch Health 2012;82(5):233–8.

15. Chrisman SP, Schiff MA, Chung SK, et al. Implementation of concussion legislation and extent of concussion education for athletes, parents, and coaches in Washington State. Am J Sports Med 2014;42(5):1190–6.

16. Shenouda C, Hendrickson P, Davenport K, et al. The effects of concussion legislation one year later–what have we learned: a descriptive pilot survey of youth soccer player associates. PM R 2012;4(6):427–35.

17. Williamson RW, Gerhardstein D, Cardenas J, et al. Concussion 101: the current state of concussion education programs. Neurosurgery 2014;75(Suppl 4):S131–5.

18. Chrisman SP, Quitiquit C, Rivara FP. Qualitative study of barriers to concussive symptom reporting in high school athletics. J Adolesc Health 2013;52(3): 330–5.e3.

19. Rivara FP, Schiff MA, Chrisman SP, et al. The effect of coach education on reporting of concussions among high school athletes after passage of a concussion law. Am J Sports Med 2014;42(5):1197–203.

20. O'Kane JW, Levy MR, Neradilek M, et al. Evaluation of the zachery lystedt law among female youth soccer players. Phys Sportsmed 2014;42(3):39–44.

21. Register-Mihalik JK, Guskiewicz KM, McLeod TC, et al. Knowledge, attitude, and concussion-reporting behaviors among high school athletes: a preliminary study. J Athl Train 2013;48(5):645–53.

22. Kurowski B, Pomerantz WJ, Schaiper C, et al. Factors that influence concussion knowledge and self-reported attitudes in high school athletes. J Trauma Acute Care Surg 2014;77(3 Suppl 1):S12–7.

23. Carl RL, Kinsella SB. Pediatricians' knowledge of current sports concussion legislation and guidelines and comfort with sports concussion management: a cross-sectional study. Clin Pediatr (Phila) 2014;53(7):689–97.

24. Centers for disease control and prevention. HEADS UP. Available at: http://www.cdc.gov/headsup/index.html. Accessed September 7, 2015.

25. Centers for disease control and prevention. HEADS UP online training courses. Available at: http://www.cdc.gov/headsup/resources/training.html. Accessed September 7, 2015.

26. The National Federation of State High School Associations: concussion in sports. Available at: http://nfhslearn.com/courses/61037. Accessed September 7, 2015.

27. Gibson TB, Herring SA, Kutcher JS, et al. Analyzing the effect of state legislation on health care utilization for children with concussion. JAMA Pediatr 2015;169(2): 163–8.

28. Aubry M, Cantu R, Dvorak J, et al. Summary and agreement statement of the first international conference on concussion in sport, Vienna 2001. Recommendations for the improvement of safety and health of athletes who may suffer concussive injuries. Br J Sports Med 2002;36(1):6–10.

29. Harvey HH. Reducing traumatic brain injuries in youth sports: youth sports traumatic brain injury state laws, January 2009-December 2012. Am J Public Health 2013;103(7):1249–54.
30. Connecticut substitute house bill no. 5113. Available at: https://www.cga.ct.gov/2014/ACT/PA/2014PA-00066-R00HB-05113-PA.htm. Accessed November 1, 2015.
31. Pennsylvania senate bill 2000. Available at: http://www.legis.state.pa.us/CFDOCS/Legis/PN/Public/btCheck.cfm?txtType=PDF&sessYr=2011&sessInd=0&billBody=S&billTyp=B&billNbr=0200&pn=1637. Accessed November 1, 2015.
32. Tomei KL, Doe C, Prestigiacomo CJ, et al. Comparative analysis of state-level concussion legislation and review of current practices in concussion. Neurosurg Focus 2012;33(6):E11, 1–9.
33. Kirschen MP, Tsou A, Nelson SB, et al. Legal and ethical implications in the evaluation and management of sports-related concussion. Neurology 2014;83(4):352–8.
34. Alaska house bill 15. Available at: http://www.legis.state.ak.us/basis/get_bill_text.asp?hsid=HB0015A&session=27. Accessed November 11, 2015.
35. Alabama house bill 308. Available at: http://arc-sos.state.al.us/PAC/SOSACPDF.001/A0009329.PDF. Accessed November 11, 2015.
36. Arizona senate bill 1521. Available at: http://www.azleg.gov/legtext/50leg/1r/bills/sb1521s.pdf. Accessed November 11, 2015.
37. Colorado senate bill 11-040 jake snakenberg youth concussion act. Available at: http://www.leg.state.co.us/clics/clics2011a/csl.nsf/fsbillcont3/A9CE9CEE12645CAA8725780800800D80?open&file=040_enr.pdf. Accessed November 11, 2015.
38. Delaware State Bill 111. Available at: http://www.legis.delaware.gov/LIS/lis146.nsf/vwLegislation/SB+111/$file/legis.html?open. Accessed November 11, 2015.
39. Delaware Senate Amendment 1 Available at: http://www.legis.delaware.gov/LIS/lis146.nsf/vwlegislation/SA%201%20to%20SB%20111?opendocument. Accessed November 11, 2015.
40. Florida house bill 291. Available at: http://laws.flrules.org/files/Ch_2012-167.pdf. Accessed November 14, 2015.
41. Georgia house bill 284. Available at: http://www.legis.ga.gov/Legislation/20132014/136573.pdf. Accessed November 11, 2015.
42. Iowa Acts, Chapter 32. Available at: https://www.legis.iowa.gov/DOCS/IowaActs/84/1/pdf/Chapter_0032.pdf. Accessed November 11, 2015.
43. Kansas house bill 2182, Section 17. Available at: http://www.kslegislature.org/li_2012/b2011_12/year1/measures/documents/hb2182_enrolled.pdf. Accessed November 11, 2015.
44. Massachusetts Senate Bill 2469. Available at: https://malegislature.gov/Laws/SessionLaws/Acts/2010/Chapter166. Accessed November 11, 2015.
45. Missouri house bill 300, 334, and 387. Available at: http://www.house.mo.gov/billtracking/bills111/billpdf/truly/HB0300T.PDF. Accessed November 11, 2015.
46. Mississippi house bill 48. Available at: http://billstatus.ls.state.ms.us/documents/2014/pdf/HB/0001-0099/HB0048SG.pdf. Accessed November 11, 2015.
47. Nebraska legislative bill 260. Available at: http://www.nebraskalegislature.gov/FloorDocs/102/PDF/Slip/LB260.pdf. Accessed November 11, 2015.
48. New Hampshire Senate Bill 402. Available at: http://www.gencourt.state.nh.us/legislation/2012/SB0402.pdf. Accessed November 11, 2015.
49. New Hampshire House Bill 1113 Amended. Available at: https://legiscan.com/NH/text/HB1113/id/988881. Accessed November 11, 2015.

50. New Mexico senate bill 0001. Available at: http://www.nmlegis.gov/Sessions/10%20Regular/final/SB0001.pdf. Accessed November 11, 2015.

51. Nevada house bill 1113. Available at: http://www.ncsl.org/research/health/traumatic-brain-injury-legislation.aspx. Accessed November 11, 2015.

52. New York senate bill 3953. Available at: http://assembly.state.ny.us/leg/?default_fld=&bn=S03953&term=2011&Summary=Y&Text=Y. Accessed November 11, 2015.

53. Ohio house bill 143. Available at: http://www.lsc.ohio.gov/analyses129/12-hb143-129.pdf. Accessed November 11, 2015.

54. Oklahoma senate bill 1700. Available at: https://www.sos.ok.gov/documents/legislation/52nd/2010/2R/SB/1700.pdf. Accessed November 11, 2015.

55. Oregon senate bill 348. Available at: https://www.oregonlegislature.gov/bills_laws/lawsstatutes/2009orLaw0661.html. Accessed November 11, 2015.

56. Rhode Island house bill 5540. Available at: http://webserver.rilin.state.ri.us/PublicLaws/law11/law11237.htm. Accessed November 11, 2015. (Amended from House Bill 7036).

57. South Carolina house bill 3061. Available at: http://www.scstatehouse.gov/sess120_2013-2014/bills/3061.htm. Accessed November 11, 2015.

58. Tennessee senate bill 882. Available at: http://www.capitol.tn.gov/Bills/108/Bill/SB0882.pdf. Accessed November 14, 2015.

59. Texas house bill 2038. Available at: http://www.capitol.state.tx.us/tlodocs/82R/billtext/pdf/HB02038F.pdf#navpanes=0. Accessed November 11, 2015.

60. Utah health code Chapter 53. Available at: http://le.utah.gov/xcode/Title26/Chapter53/26-53-S301.html. Accessed November 11, 2015.

61. Virginia student athlete protection act. Available at: http://www.doe.virginia.gov/boe/guidance/health/2015_guidelines_concussions_in_student_athletes.pdf. Accessed November 1, 2015.

62. Wisconsin ACT 172. Available at: https://docs.legis.wisconsin.gov/2011/related/acts/172.pdf. Accessed November 14, 2015.

63. Louisiana senate bill 189. Act 314. Available at: http://www.legis.la.gov/legis/ViewDocument.aspx?d=760519&n=SB189%20Act%20314. Accessed November 11, 2015.

64. Vermont Act 68. Available at: http://www.leg.state.vt.us/docs/2014/Acts/ACT068.pdf. Accessed November 11, 2015.

65. Illinois public act 099-0245. Available at: http://www.ilga.gov/legislation/publicacts/fulltext.asp?Name=099-0245. Accessed November 11, 2015.

66. California education code. Available at: http://leginfo.legislature.ca.gov/faces/codes_displaySection.xhtml?lawCode=EDC&sectionNum=49475. Accessed September 26, 2015.

67. West virginia senate bill 336. Available at: http://www.legis.state.wv.us/Bill_Text_HTML/2013_SESSIONS/RS/pdf_bills/SB336%20SUB2%20ENR%20PRINTED.pdf. Accessed November 11, 2015.

68. Lowrey KM. State laws addressing youth sports-related traumatic brain injury and the future of concussion law and policy. J Bus & Tech L 2014;10(1):61–72.

69. Arkansas concussion protocol act. Available at: http://www.arkleg.state.ar.us/assembly/2013/2013R/Acts/Act1435.pdf. Accessed September 26, 2015.

70. New jersey senate bill 2275. Available at: http://www.njleg.state.nj.us/2014/Bills/S2500/2275_I1.HTM. Accessed September 26, 2015.

71. Nebraska revised statutes chapter 71-9104. Available at: http://nebraskalegislature.gov/laws/statutes.php?statute=71-9104&print=true. Accessed September 26, 2015.

72. California education code AB-2127. Available at: http://leginfo.legislature.ca.gov/faces/billNavClient.xhtml?bill_id=201320140AB2127. Accessed September 26, 2015.
73. Institute of Medicine (IOM), National Research Council (NRC). Sports-related concussions in youth: improving the science, changing the culture. Washington, DC: The National Academies Press; 2013.
74. Bompadre V, Jinguji TM, Yanez ND, et al. Washington state's lystedt law in concussion documentation in seattle public high schools. J Athl Train 2014; 49(4):486–92.
75. Morrissey D, Raukar NP, Andrade-Koziol J, et al. Statewide assessment of the rhode island school and youth programs concussion act. J Trauma Acute Care Surg 2014;77(3 Suppl 1):S8–11.

Index

Note: Page numbers of article titles are in **boldface** type.

A

Activity restrictions
    after concussion in athletes, **487–501** (See also Concussion; Sports-related concussion
        (SRC))
Aerobic exercise therapy
    in PCS rehabilitation, 446
β-Amyloid
    in CTE, 507–508
Athlete(s)
    concussion in (See Sports-related concussion (SRC))
    legislation on SRC effects on
        education, 514–515
    PCS in
        nonpharmacologic approaches in recovery from, 442
    pediatric
        activity restrictions following SRC in, 494–495
Axonal injury
    concussion and, 378–380

B

Balance error scoring system (BESS)
    in concussion in athletes sideline management, 400–402
BCTT. See Buffalo Concussion Treadmill Test (BCTT)
BESS. See Balance error scoring system (BESS)
Biomarker(s)
    of CTE, 505
Brain injury
    traumatic (See Traumatic brain injury (TBI))
Buffalo Concussion Treadmill Test (BCTT)
    in PCS rehabilitation, 446–448

C

Cerebral blood flow
    concussion and, 377–378
Children
    SRC in
        activity restrictions following, 494–495
Chronic traumatic encephalopathy (CTE)
    concussion and, **503–511**

Phys Med Rehabil Clin N Am 27 (2016) 529–537
http://dx.doi.org/10.1016/S1047-9651(16)30008-0
1047-9651/16/$ – see front matter © 2016 Elsevier Inc. All rights reserved.

V

Moving?

Make sure your subscription moves with you!

To notify us of your new address, find your **Clinics Account Number** (located on your mailing label above your name), and contact customer service at:

Email: journalscustomerservice-usa@elsevier.com

800-654-2452 (subscribers in the U.S. & Canada)
314-447-8871 (subscribers outside of the U.S. & Canada)

Fax number: 314-447-8029

Elsevier Health Sciences Division
Subscription Customer Service
3251 Riverport Lane
Maryland Heights, MO 63043

*To ensure uninterrupted delivery of your subscription, please notify us at least 4 weeks in advance of move.

Printed and bound by CPI Group (UK) Ltd, Croydon, CR0 4YY

03/10/2024

01040394-0014